Facts

made

Incredibly Quick!™

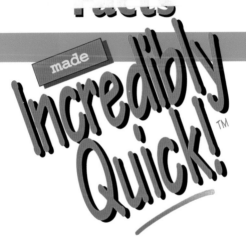

Waterproof and Washable
Write on the pages with a ballpoint pen.
Remove old information with an
alcohol wipe and reuse!

LIPPINCOTT WILLIAMS & WILKINS
A **Wolters Kluwer** Company

Philadelphia · Baltimore · New York · London
Buenos Aires · Hong Kong · Sydney · Tokyo

Staff

Executive Publisher
Judith A. Schilling McCann, RN, MSN

Editorial Director
David Moreau

Clinical Director
Joan M. Robinson, RN, MSN

Senior Art Director
Arlene Putterman

Art Director
Mary Ludwicki

Editorial Project Manager
Jaime Stockslager Buss, ELS

Clinical Project Manager
Beverly Ann Tscheschlog, RN, BS

Editors
Rita Breedlove, Brenna H. Mayer

Clinical Editor
Jana L. Sciarra, RN, MSN, CRNP

Copy Editors
Kimberly Bilotta (supervisor), Amy Furman,
Pamela Wingrod

Designer
Lynn Foulk

Illustrator
Bot Roda

Digital Composition Services
Diane Paluba (manager), Joyce Rossi Biletz

Manufacturing
Patricia K. Dorshaw (director), Beth J. Welsh

Editorial Assistants
Megan L. Aldinger, Karen J. Kirk,
Linda K. Ruhf

Indexer
Jaime Stockslager Buss, ELS

PEDMIQ010106—060409
ISBN-13: 978-1-58255-993-3
ISBN-10: 1-58255-993-7

Growth & development

Theories of development, Growth rates, Height and weight tables, Stages of development, Sexual maturity, Preparation for hospitalization and surgery

Assessment

Preventive care, Health history, Vital signs, Length and head circumference, Physical examination, Dentition, Pain assessment, Burns, Mental health, Abuse

Laboratory values

Chemistry tests, CBC, Antibiotic levels, Urine, Acid-base disorders

Meds/IV therapy

Immunization schedules, Calculations, Conversions, BSA, Administration methods and sites, Fluid needs, I.V. solutions, Blood compatibility, Insulin

Emergency

CPR, Choking, ACLS algorithms

Teaching

SIDS, Choking, Toileting, Burns, Poison, Drowning, Falls, Vehicle safety

Resources

Conversion, Nutrition, Sleep, Cultural concerns, Eng-Span guide

Common abbreviations

ABG	arterial blood gas
AED	automated external defibrillator
ALT	alanine aminotransferase
AST	aspartate aminotransferase
BP	blood pressure
BSA	body surface area
BUN	blood urea nitrogen
C	Celsius
cm	centimeter
CO₂	carbon dioxide
CPR	cardiopulmonary resuscitation
DTaP	diphtheria and tetanus toxoids and acellular pertussis
ECG	electrocardiogram
ESR	erythrocyte sedimentation rate
F	Fahrenheit
FSH	follicle-stimulating hormone
g	gram
G	gauge
GGT	gamma-glutamyltransferase
GI	gastrointestinal
GU	genitourinary
HBsAg	hepatitis B surface antigen
HBV	hepatitis B vaccine
HCO₃	bicarbonate
HDL	high-density lipoprotein
Hib	*Haemophilus influenzae* type B
HIV	human immunodeficiency virus
HR	heart rate
I.M.	intramuscular
IPV	inactivated poliovirus vaccine
I.V.	intravenous
kcal	kilocalorie
kg	kilogram
L	liter
lb	pound
LDL	low-density lipoprotein
LH	luteinizing hormone
LOC	level of consciousness
mcg	microgram
mEq	milliequivalent
mg	milligram
ml	milliliter
MMR	measles, mumps, rubella
NaCl	sodium chloride
oz	ounce
PALS	pediatric advanced life support
PCV	pneumococcal conjugate vaccine
PKU	phenylketonuria
P.O.	by mouth
PPV	pneumococcal polysaccharide vaccine
RBC	red blood cell
SIDS	sudden infant death syndrome
STD	sexually transmitted disease
tbs	tablespoon
Td	tetanus toxoid
TSH	thyroid-stimulating hormone
tsp	teaspoon
VZV	varicella zoster vaccine
WBC	white blood cell

Stages of childhood development

- *Infancy:* Birth to age 1
- *Toddler stage:* Ages 1 to 3
- *Preschool stage:* Ages 3 to 6
- *School-age:* Ages 6 to 12
- *Adolescence:* Ages 12 to 19

Patterns of development

This chart shows the patterns of development and their progression and gives examples of each.

Pattern	Path of progression	Examples
Cephalocaudal	From head to toe	Head control precedes ability to walk.
Proximodistal	From the trunk to the tips of the extremities	The young infant can move his arms and legs but can't pick up objects with his fingers.
General to specific	From simple tasks to more complex tasks (mastering simple tasks before advancing to those that are more complex)	The child progresses from crawling to walking to skipping.

Theories of development

The child development theories discussed in this chart shouldn't be compared directly because they measure different aspects of development. Erik Erikson's psychosocial-based theory is the most commonly accepted model for child development, although it can't be empirically tested.

Age-group	Psychosocial theory	Cognitive theory	Psychosexual theory	Moral development theory
Infancy (birth to age 1)	Trust versus mistrust	Sensorimotor (birth to age 2)	Oral	Not applicable
Toddlerhood (ages 1 to 3)	Autonomy versus shame and doubt	Sensorimotor to pre-operational	Anal	Preconventional
Preschool age (ages 3 to 6)	Initiative versus guilt	Preoperational (ages 2 to 7)	Phallic	Preconventional
School age (ages 6 to 12)	Industry versus inferiority	Concrete operational (ages 7 to 11)	Latency	Conventional
Adolescence (ages 12 to 19)	Identity versus role confusion	Formal operational thought (ages 11 to 15)	Genitalia	Postconventional

A closer look at theories of development

Psychosocial theory (Erik Erikson)

• Trust versus mistrust: Develops trust as the primary caregiver meets his needs.
• Autonomy versus shame and doubt: Learns to control body functions; becomes increasingly independent.
• Initiative versus guilt: Learns about the world through play; develops a conscience.
• Industry versus inferiority: Enjoys working with others; tends to follow rules; forming social relationships takes on greater importance.
• Identity versus role confusion: Is preoccupied with how he looks and how others view him; tries to establish his own identity while meeting the expectations of his peers.

Cognitive theory (Jean Piaget)

• Sensorimotor stage: Progresses from reflex activity, through simple repetitive behaviors, to imitative behaviors; concepts to be mastered include object permanence, causality, and spatial relationships.
• Preoperational stage: Is egocentric and employs magical thinking; concepts to be mastered include representational language and symbols and transductive reasoning.
• Concrete operational stage: Thought processes become more logical and coherent; can't think abstractly; concepts to be mastered include sorting, ordering, and classifying facts to use in problem solving.
• Formal operational thought stage: Is adaptable and flexible; concepts to be mastered include abstract ideas and concepts, possibilities, inductive reasoning, and complex deductive reasoning.

Psychosexual theory (Sigmund Freud)

• Involves the *id* (primitive instincts; requires immediate gratification), *ego* (conscious, rational part of the personality), and *superego* (a person's conscience and ideals).
• Oral stage: Seeks pleasure through sucking, biting, and other oral activities.
• Anal stage: Goes through toilet training, learning how to control his excreta.
• Phallic stage: Interested in his genitalia; discovers the difference between boys and girls.

(continued)

A closer look at theories of development

(continued)

• Latency period: Concentrates on playing and learning (not focused on a particular body area).
• Genitalia stage: At maturation of the reproductive system, develops the capacity for object love and maturity.

Moral development theory (Lawrence Kohlberg)

• Preconventional level of morality: Attempts to follow rules set by authority figures; adjusts behavior according to good and bad, right and wrong.
• Conventional level of morality: Seeks conformity and loyalty; follows fixed rules; attempts to maintain social order.
• Postconventional autonomous level of morality: Strives to construct a value system independent of authority figures and peers.

Expected growth rates

Age-group	Weight	Height or length	Head circumference
Infancy (birth to age 1)	• Birth weight doubles by age 5 months • Birth weight triples by age 1 • Gains 1½ lb (680 g)/month for first 5 months • Gains ¾ lb (340 g)/month during second 6 months	• Birth length increases by 50% by age 1, with most growth occurring in the trunk rather than the legs during the first 3 months • Grows 1″ (2.5 cm)/month during first 6 months • Grows ½″ (1.3 cm)/month during second 6 months	• Increases by almost 33% by age 1 • Increases ¾″ (2 cm)/month during the first 3 months • Increases ⅓″ (1 cm)/month from ages 4 to 6 months • Increases ¼″ (0.5 cm)/month during second 6 months
Toddlerhood (ages 1 to 3)	• Birth weight quadruples by age 2½ • Gains 8 oz (227 g)/month from ages 1 to 2 • Gains 3 to 5 lb (1.5 to 2.5 kg) from ages 2 to 3	• Growth occurs mostly in legs rather than trunk • Grows 3½″ to 5″ (9 to 12.5 cm) from ages 1 to 2 • Grows 2″ to 2½″ (5 to 6.5 cm) from ages 2 to 3	• Increases 1″ from ages 1 to 2 • Increases less than ½″ (1.3 cm)/year from ages 2 to 3
Preschool age (ages 3 to 6)	• Gains 3 to 5 lb (1.5 to 2.5 kg)/year	• Growth occurs mostly in legs rather than trunk • Grows 2½″ to 3″ (6.5 to 7.5 cm)/year	• Increases less than ½″/year from ages 3 to 5
School age (ages 6 to 12)	• Gains 6 lb (2.5 kg)/year	• Grows 2″ (5 cm)/year	• Not applicable
Adolescence (ages 12 to 19)	• Girls: Gain 15 to 55 lb (7 to 25 kg) • Boys: Gain 15 to 65 lb (7 to 30 kg)	• Girls: Grow 3″ to 6″ (7.5 to 15 cm)/year until age 16 • Boys: Grow 3″ to 6″/year until age 18	• Not applicable

Height measurements for boys, ages 2 through 18 years

Age	Height by percentiles					
	10%		50%		90%	
	cm	inches	cm	inches	cm	inches
2 years	84.7	33.4	91.0	35.8	97.6	38.4
3 years	92.5	36.4	98.8	38.9	103.9	40.9
4 years	100.7	39.6	106.5	41.9	112.1	44.1
5 years	105.8	41.7	114.2	45.0	119.1	46.9
6 years	111.6	43.9	119.3	47.0	125.9	49.6
7 years	117.7	46.4	126.6	49.8	135.0	53.2
8 years	123.8	48.7	132.5	52.1	140.9	55.5
9 years	130.1	51.2	137.5	54.1	145.4	57.3
10 years	133.4	52.5	141.1	55.6	149.1	58.7
11 years	139.7	55.0	148.8	58.6	157.4	62.0
12 years	143.0	56.3	153.9	60.6	167.8	66.0
13 years	147.2	58.0	160.5	63.2	171.6	67.6
14 years	155.1	61.1	169.1	66.6	179.0	70.5
15 years	163.5	64.4	174.2	68.6	183.4	72.2
16 years	166.6	65.6	175.6	69.1	182.8	72.0
17 years	165.7	65.2	175.3	69.0	184.2	72.5
18 years	168.1	66.2	176.1	69.3	184.9	72.8

Adapted from McDowell, M.A., et al. *Anthropometric Reference Data for Children and Adults: U.S. Population, 1999-2002.* U.S. Department of Health and Human Services, Centers for Disease Control and Prevention, National Center for Health Statistics, 2005.

Weight measurements for boys, ages 1 through 18 years

| Age | Weight by percentiles | | | | | |
| | 10% | | 50% | | 90% | |
	kg	lb	kg	lb	kg	lb
1 year	9.5	20.9	11.1	24.4	13.1	28.8
2 years	11.5	25.3	13.7	30.1	15.9	35.2
3 years	12.9	28.4	16.0	35.2	18.8	41.4
4 years	15.4	34.0	18.2	40.2	21.4	47.1
5 years	17.0	37.5	20.7	45.7	26.0	57.4
6 years	18.2	40.1	22.7	50.0	29.0	63.9
7 years	21.6	47.6	25.7	56.7	33.1	72.9
8 years	23.5	51.7	30.4	66.9	45.8	100.9
9 years	26.5	58.4	34.1	75.2	49.6	109.3
10 years	27.8	61.2	36.1	79.6	50.2	110.6
11 years	31.2	68.8	42.1	92.9	57.2	126.2
12 years	35.0	77.1	46.3	102.1	71.8	158.3
13 years	34.2	75.4	53.0	116.9	75.3	166.1
14 years	45.4	100.0	61.0	134.5	90.1	198.7
15 years	51.7	114.0	64.0	141.0	93.1	205.2
16 years	54.9	121.0	69.4	153.1	98.1	216.2
17 years	55.6	122.6	72.9	160.8	98.9	218.0
18 years	58.3	128.5	70.6	155.7	97.6	215.2

Adapted from McDowell, M.A., et al. *Anthropometric Reference Data for Children and Adults: U.S. Population, 1999-2002.* U.S. Department of Health and Human Services, Centers for Disease Control and Prevention, National Center for Health Statistics, 2005.

Height measurements for girls, ages 2 through 18 years

| Age | Height by percentiles | | | | | |
| | 10% | | 50% | | 90% | |
	cm	inches	cm	inches	cm	inches
2 years	84.9	33.4	89.7	35.3	95.3	37.5
3 years	92.6	36.4	98.1	38.6	102.2	40.2
4 years	100.3	39.5	105.8	41.6	111.7	44.0
5 years	106.5	41.9	111.9	44.0	119.5	47.1
6 years	110.2	43.4	117.2	46.1	124.0	48.8
7 years	117.5	46.3	124.2	48.9	131.6	51.8
8 years	123.0	48.4	131.0	51.6	138.5	54.5
9 years	128.2	50.5	137.2	54.0	146.5	57.7
10 years	*	*	142.8	56.2	*	*
11 years	141.1	55.6	151.3	59.6	161.1	63.4
12 years	146.5	57.7	156.6	61.7	164.8	64.9
13 years	149.9	59.0	158.4	62.3	168.6	66.4
14 years	154.1	60.7	161.6	63.6	169.2	66.6
15 years	153.2	60.3	162.5	64.0	169.3	66.7
16 years	154.0	60.6	161.3	63.5	169.6	66.8
17 years	154.6	60.9	163.5	64.4	172.1	67.8
18 years	155.4	61.2	163.1	64.2	171.2	67.4

* Figure doesn't meet standard of reliability or precision.

Adapted from McDowell, M.A., et al. *Anthropometric Reference Data for Children and Adults: U.S. Population, 1999-2002.* U.S. Department of Health and Human Services, Centers for Disease Control and Prevention, National Center for Health Statistics, 2005.

Weight measurements for girls, ages 1 through 18 years

| Age | Weight by percentiles | | | | | |
	10%		50%		90%	
	kg	lb	kg	lb	kg	lb
1 year	9.1	20.0	10.6	23.4	12.9	28.4
2 years	11.1	24.5	12.9	28.4	15.6	34.3
3 years	12.9	28.4	15.0	33.2	17.5	38.6
4 years	14.7	32.4	17.2	38.0	20.8	46.0
5 years	16.6	36.6	19.2	42.3	26.9	59.4
6 years	17.9	39.5	21.5	47.3	27.7	61.0
7 years	20.3	44.7	24.7	54.4	32.9	72.5
8 years	22.3	49.3	29.1	64.1	44.1	97.3
9 years	25.6	56.5	34.1	75.2	48.4	106.7
10 years	27.8	61.3	38.3	84.5	53.9	118.9
11 years	32.9	72.6	44.9	98.9	69.0	152.2
12 years	36.3	80.1	49.7	109.6	69.3	152.7
13 years	41.0	90.4	55.5	122.4	79.7	175.6
14 years	46.2	101.8	56.3	124.1	80.9	178.4
15 years	45.7	100.8	57.6	126.9	83.3	183.6
16 years	47.7	105.3	59.1	130.3	84.1	185.5
17 years	46.7	102.9	59.3	130.8	77.3	170.3
18 years	47.0	103.6	60.9	134.3	93.2	205.5

Adapted from McDowell, M.A., et al. *Anthropometric Reference Data for Children and Adults: U.S. Population, 1999-2002.* U.S. Department of Health and Human Services, Centers for Disease Control and Prevention, National Center for Health Statistics, 2005.

Infant gross and fine motor development

Age	Gross motor skills	Fine motor skills
1 month	• Can hold head parallel momentarily but still has marked head lag • Back is rounded in sitting position, with no head control	• Strong grasp reflex • Hands remain mostly closed in a fist
2 months	• In prone position, can lift head 45 degrees off table • In sitting position, back is still rounded but with more head control	• Diminishing grasp reflex • Hands open more often
3 months	• Displays only slight head lag when pulled to a seated position • In prone position, can use forearms to lift head and shoulders 45 to 90 degrees off table • Can bear slight amount of weight on legs in standing position	• Grasp reflex now absent • Hands remain open • Can hold a rattle and clutch own hand
4 months	• No head lag • Holds head erect in sitting position, back less rounded • In prone position, can lift head and chest 90 degrees off table • Can roll from back to side	• Regards own hand • Can grasp objects with both hands • May try to reach for an object without success • Can move objects toward mouth
5 months	• No head lag • Holds head erect and steady when sitting • Back is straight • Can put feet to mouth when supine • Can roll from stomach to back	• Can voluntarily grasp objects • Can move objects directly to mouth

Infant gross and fine motor development
(continued)

Age	Gross motor skills	Fine motor skills
6 months	• Can lift chest and upper abdomen off table, bearing weight on hands • Can roll from back to stomach • Can bear almost all of weight on feet when held in standing position • Sits with support	• Can hold bottle • Can voluntarily grasp and release objects
7 months	• Can sit, leaning forward on hands for support • When in standing position, can bear full weight on legs and bounce	• Transfers objects from hand to hand • Rakes at objects • Can bang objects on table
8 months	• Can sit alone without assistance • Can move from sitting to kneeling position	• Has beginning pincer grasp • Reaches for objects out of reach
9 months	• Creeps on hands and knees with belly off floor • Pulls to standing position • Can stand, holding on to furniture	• Refining pincer grasp • Use of dominant hand evident
10 months	• Can move from prone to sitting position • Stands with support; may lift a foot as if to take a step	• Refining pincer grasp
11 months	• Can cruise (take side steps while holding on to furniture) or walk with both hands held	• Can move objects into containers • Deliberately drops object to have it picked up • Neat pincer grasp
12 months	• Cruises well, may walk with one hand held • May try to stand alone	• May attempt to build a two-block tower • Can crudely turn pages of a book • Feeds self with cup and spoon

Infant language and social development

Age	Behaviors
0 to 2 months	• Listens to voices; quiets to soft music, singing, or talking • Distinguishes mother's voice after 1 week, father's by 2 weeks • Prefers human voices to other sounds • Produces vowel sounds "ah," "eh," and "oh"
3 to 4 months	• Coos and gurgles • Babbles in response to someone talking to him • Babbles for own pleasure with giggles, shrieks, and laughs • Says "da," "ba," "ma," "pa," and "ga" • Vocalizes more to a real person than to a picture • Responds to caregiver with social smile by 3 months
5 to 6 months	• Notices how his speech influences actions of others • Makes "raspberries" and smacks lips • Begins learning to take turns in conversation • Talks to toys and self in mirror • Recognizes names and familiar sounds
7 to 9 months	• Tries to imitate more sounds; makes several sounds in one breath • Begins learning the meaning of "no" by tone of voice and actions • Experiences early literacy; enjoys listening to simple books being read • Enjoys pat-a-cake • Recognizes and responds to his name and names of familiar objects
10 to 12 months	• May have a few word approximations, such as "bye-bye" and "hi" • Follows one-step instructions such as "go to daddy" • Recognizes words as symbols for objects • Says "ma-ma-ma" and "da-da-da"

Infant cognitive development and play

This chart shows the infant's development of two cognitive skills, object permanence and causality. It includes play, an integral part of infant development.

Age	Object permanence	Causality	Play
0 to 4 months	• Objects out of sight are out of mind • Continues to look at hand after object is dropped out of it	• Creates bodily sensations by actions (for example, thumb-sucking)	• Grasps and moves objects such as a rattle • Looks at contrasting colors
4 to 8 months	• Can locate a partially hidden object • Visually tracks objects when dropped	• Uses causal behaviors to re-create accidentally discovered interesting effects (for example, kicking the bed after the chance discovery that this will set in motion a mobile above the bed)	• Reaches and grasps an object and then will mouth, shake, bang, and drop the object (in this order)
9 to 12 months	• Object permanence develops • Can find an object when hidden but can't retrieve an object that's moved in plain view from one hiding place to another • Knows parent still exists when out of view but can't imagine where they might be (separation anxiety may arise)	• Understanding of cause and effect leads to intentional behavior aimed at getting specific results	• Manipulates objects to inspect with eyes and hands • Has ability to process information simultaneously instead of sequentially • Ability to play peek-a-boo demonstrates object permanence

Toddler gross and fine motor development

Age	Gross motor skills	Fine motor skills
1 year	• Walks alone using a wide stance • Begins to run but falls easily	• Grasps a very small object (but can't release it until about 15 months)
2 years	• Runs without falling most of the time • Throws a ball overhand without losing his balance • Jumps with both feet • Walks up and down stairs • Uses push and pull toys	• Builds a tower of four blocks • Scribbles on paper • Drops a small pellet into a small, narrow container • Uses a spoon well and drinks well from a covered cup • Undresses himself

Toddler language development

During toddlerhood, the ability to understand speech is much more developed than the ability to speak. This chart highlights language development during the toddler years.

Age	Language skills
1 year	• The toddler uses one-word sentences or holophrases (real words that are meant to represent entire phrases or ideas). • The toddler has learned about four words. • About 25% of a 1-year-old's vocalization is understandable.
2 years	• The number of words learned has increased from about 4 (at age 1) to approximately 300. • The toddler uses multiword (two- to three-word) sentences. • About 65% of speech is understandable. • Frequent, repetitive naming of objects helps toddlers learn appropriate words for objects.

Toddler socialization

Toddlers develop social skills that determine the way they interact with others. As the toddler develops psychologically, he can:
• differentiate himself from others
• tolerate being separated from a parent
• withstand delayed gratification
• control his bodily functions
• acquire socially acceptable behaviors
• communicate verbally
• become less egocentric.

Toddler psychosocial development

According to Erikson, the developmental task of toddlerhood is autonomy versus doubt and shame. Toddlers:
• are in the final stages of developing a sense of trust (the task from infancy) and start asserting control, independence, and autonomy
• display negativism in their quest for autonomy
• need to maintain sameness and reliability for comfort; employ ritualism
• view "paternal" person in their life as a significant other
• develop an ego, which creates conflict between the impulses of the id (which requires immediate gratification) and socially acceptable actions
• begin to develop a superego, or conscience, which starts to incorporate the morals of society.

Toddler cognitive development

According to Piaget, a child moves from the sensorimotor stage of infancy and early toddlerhood (birth to age 2) to the longer, preoperational stage (ages 2 to 7). In these stages, toddlers:
• employ tertiary circular reactions (use of active experimentation; also called *trial and error* [in the 13- to 18-month old])
• may be aware of the relationship between two events (cause and effect) but may be unable to transfer that knowledge to a new situation
• look for new ways to accomplish tasks through mental calculations (ages 18 to 24 months)
• advance in understanding object permanence and gain awareness of the existence of objects or people that are out of sight
• engage in imitative play, which indicates a deeper understanding of their role in the family
• begin to use preoperational thought with increasing use of words as symbols, problem solving, and creative thinking.

Toddler play

- Play changes considerably as the toddler's motor skills develop; he uses his physical skills to push and pull objects; to climb up, down, in, and out; and to run or ride on toys.
- A short attention span requires frequent changes in toys and play media.
- Toddlers increase their cognitive abilities by manipulating objects and learning about their qualities, which makes tactile play (with water, sand, finger paints, clay) important.
- Many play activities involve imitating behaviors the child sees at home, which helps them learn new actions and skills.
- Toddlers engage in parallel play—playing with others without actually interacting. In this type of play, children play side-by-side, commonly with similar objects. Interaction is limited to the occasional comment or trading of toys.

Safe toddler toys

- Play dough and modeling clay
- Building blocks
- Plastic, pretend housekeeping toys, such as pots, pans, and play food
- Stackable rings and blocks of varying sizes
- Toy telephones
- Wooden puzzles with big pieces
- Textured or cloth books
- Plastic musical instruments and noise-makers
- Toys that roll, such as cars and trains
- Tricycle or riding car
- Fat crayons and coloring books
- Stuffed animals with painted faces (button eyes are a choking hazard)

Preschool gross and fine motor development

Age	Gross motor skills	Fine motor skills
3 years	• Stands on one foot for a few seconds • Climbs stairs with alternating feet • Jumps in place • Performs a broad jump • Dances but with somewhat poor balance • Kicks a ball • Rides a tricycle	• Builds a tower of 9 to 10 blocks and a 3-block bridge • Copies a circle and imitates a cross and vertical and horizontal lines • Draws a circle as a head, but not a complete stick figure • Uses a fork well
4 years	• Hops, jumps, and skips on one foot • Throws a ball overhand • Rides a tricycle or bicycle with training wheels	• Copies a square and traces a cross • Draws recognizable familiar objects or human figures
5 years	• Skips, using alternate feet • Jumps rope • Balances on each foot for 4 to 5 seconds	• Copies a triangle and a diamond • Draws a stick figure with several body parts, including facial features

Preschool psychosocial development

According to Erikson, children ages 3 to 5 have mastered a sense of autonomy and face the task of initiative versus guilt. During this time, the child's:
• significant other is the family
• conscience begins to develop, introducing the concept of right and wrong
• sense of guilt arises when he feels that his imagination and activities are unacceptable or clash with his parents' expectations
• simple reasoning develops and longer periods of delayed gratification are tolerated.

Preschool language development and socialization

By the time a child reaches preschool age:
• his vocabulary increases to about 900 words by age 3 and 2,100 words by age 5
• he may talk incessantly and ask many "why" questions
• he usually talks in three- to four-word sentences by age 3; by age 5, he speaks in longer sentences that contain all parts of speech.

Socialization continues to develop as the preschooler's world expands beyond himself and his family (although parents remain central). Regular interaction with same-age children is necessary to further develop social skills.

Preschool play

In the preschool stage, the parallel play of toddlerhood is replaced by more interactive, cooperative play, including:
• more associative play, in which children play together
• better understanding of the concept of sharing
• enjoyment of large motor activities, such as swinging, riding tricycles or bicycles, and throwing balls
• more dramatic play, in which the child lives out the dramas of human life (in preschool years) and may have imaginary playmates.

Preschool cognitive development

Piaget's theory divides the preoperational phase of the preschool years into two stages.

Preconceptual phase

During the preconceptual phase (from ages 2 to 4), the child can:
• form beginning concepts that aren't as complete or logical as an adult's
• make simple classifications
• rationalize specific concepts but not the idea as a whole
• exhibit egocentric thinking (evaluating each situation based on his feelings or experiences, rather than those of others).

Intuitive thought phase

During the intuitive thought phase (from ages 4 to 7), the child:
• can classify, quantify, and relate objects (but can't yet understand the principles behind these operations)
• uses intuitive thought processes (but can't fully see the viewpoints of others)
• uses many words appropriately (but without true understanding of their meaning).

Preschool moral and spiritual development

Kohlberg's preconventional phase spans the preschool years and more, extending from ages 4 to 10. During this phase:
• conscience emerges and emphasis is on control
• the preschooler's moral standards are those of others, and he understands that these standards must be followed to avoid punishment for inappropriate behavior or gain rewards for good or desired behavior
• the preschooler behaves according to what freedom is given or what restriction is placed on his actions.

Preschoolers can understand the basic plot of simple religious stories but typically don't grasp the underlying meanings. Religious principles are best learned from concrete images in picture books and small statues such as those seen at a place of worship.

During this stage, children may view an illness or hospitalization as a punishment from a higher being for some real or perceived bad behavior.

School-age fine motor development

• Development of small-muscle and eye-hand coordination increases during the school-age years, leading to the skilled handling of tools, such as pencils and papers for drawing and writing.

• During the remainder of this period, the child refines physical and motor skills and coordination.

Pubertal changes

• The pubertal growth spurt begins in girls at about age 10 and in boys at about age 12.
• The feet are the first part of the body to experience a growth spurt.
• Increased foot size is followed by a rapid increase in leg length and then trunk growth.
• In addition to bones, gonadal hormone levels increase and cause the sexual organs to mature.

Preparation for menses

• The first menstruation (called *menarche*) can occur as early as age 9 or as late as age 17 and still be considered normal.
• The menstrual cycle may be irregular at first.
• Secondary sexual characteristics may start to develop (breasts, hips, and pubic hair), and the girl may experience a sudden increase in height.

School-age language development and socialization

• The school-age child has an efficient vocabulary and begins to correct previous mistakes in usage.
• Peers become increasingly significant; his need to find his place within a group is important.

• The child may be overly concerned with peer rules; however, parental guidance continues to play an important role in his life.
• The school-age child typically has two to three best friends (although choice of friends may change frequently).

School-age psychosocial development

The school-age child enters Erikson's stage of industry versus inferiority. In this stage:
• the child wants to work and produce, accomplishing and achieving tasks
• the child may display negative attributes of inadequacy and inferiority if too much is expected of him or if he feels unable to measure up to set standards.

School-age cognitive development

The school-age child is in Piaget's concrete-operational period. In this period:
• magical thinking diminishes, and the child has a much better understanding of cause and effect
• the child begins to accept rules but may not necessarily understand them
• the child is ready for basic reading, writing, and arithmetic
• abstract thinking begins to develop during the middle elementary school years
• parents remain very important and adult reassurance of the child's competence and basic self-worth is essential.

School-age moral and spiritual development

The school-age child is in Kohlberg's conventional level. During this time, the child behaves according to socially acceptable norms because an authority figure tells him to do so. As the child approaches adolescence, school and parental authority is questioned, and even challenged or opposed. The importance of the peer group intensifies, and it eventually becomes the source of behavior standards and models.

Spiritual lessons should be taught in concrete terms during this time. Children have a hard time understanding supernatural religious symbols.

Adolescent psychosocial development

According to Erikson, adolescents enter the stage of identity versus role confusion. During this stage, they:
• experience rapid changes in their bodies
• have a preoccupation with looks and others' perceptions of them
• feel pressure to meet expectations of peers and conform to peer standards (diminishes by late adolescence as young adults become more aware of who they are)
• try to establish their own identities.

Adolescent cognitive development

Teenagers move from the concrete thinking of childhood into Piaget's stage of formal operational thought, which is characterized by:
• logical reasoning about abstract concepts
• derivation of conclusions from hypothetical premises
• forethought of future events instead of focus on the present (as in childhood).

Adolescent moral and spiritual development

Kohlberg's conventional level of moral development continues into early adolescence. At this level, adolescents do what is right because it's the socially acceptable action.

As adolescence ends, teenagers enter the postconventional, or *principled,* level of moral development. During this time, adolescents:
• form moral decisions independent of their peer group
• choose values for themselves instead of letting values be dictated by peers
• develop solidified worldviews
• formulate questions about the larger world as they considers religion, philosophy, and the values held by parents, friends, and others
• sort through and adopt religious beliefs that are consistent with their own moral character.

Development of secondary sex characteristics

The pituitary gland is stimulated at puberty to produce androgen steroids responsible for secondary sex characteristics. The hypothalamus produces gonadotropin-releasing hormone, which triggers the anterior pituitary gland to produce follicle-stimulating hormone (FSH) and luteinizing hormone (LH). FSH and LH promote testicular maturation and sperm production in boys and initiate the ovulation cycle in girls.

Male secondary sexual development

• Male secondary sexual development consists of genital growth and the appearance of pubic and body hair.
• Most boys achieve active spermatogenesis at ages 12 to 15.

Female secondary sexual development

• Female secondary sexual development involves increases in the size of the ovaries, uterus, vagina, labia, and breasts.
• The first visible sign of sexual maturity is the appearance of breast buds.
• Body hair appears in the pubic area and under the arms, and menarche occurs.
• The ovaries, present at birth, remain inactive until puberty.

Sexual maturity in boys

Genital development and pubic hair growth are the first signs of sexual maturity in boys. The illustrations below show the development of the male genitalia and pubic hair in puberty.

Stage 1
No pubic hair is present.

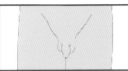

Stage 2
Downy hair develops laterally and later becomes dark; the scrotum becomes more textured, and the penis and testes may become larger.

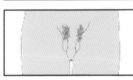

Stage 3
Pubic hair extends across the pubis; the scrotum and testes are larger; the penis elongates.

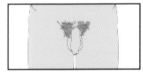

Stage 4
Pubic hair becomes more abundant and curls, and the genitalia resemble those of adults; the glans penis has become larger and broader, and the scrotum becomes darker.

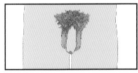

Stage 5
Pubic hair resembles an adult's in quality and pattern and the hair extends to the inner borders of the thighs; the testes and scrotum are adult in size.

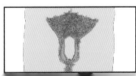

Sexual maturity in girls

Breast development and pubic hair growth are the first signs of sexual maturity in girls. These illustrations show the development of the female breast and pubic hair in puberty.

Breast development

Stage 1
Only the *papilla* (nipple) elevates (not shown).

Stage 2
Breast buds appear; the areola is slightly widened and appears as a small mound.

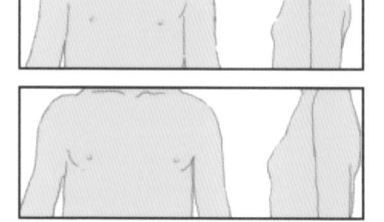

Stage 3
The entire breast enlarges; the nipple doesn't protrude.

Stage 4
The breast enlarges; the nipple and the papilla protrude and appear as a secondary mound.

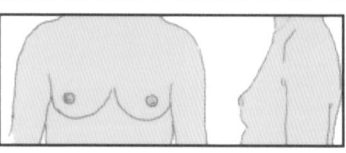

Stage 5
The adult breast has developed; the nipple protrudes and the areola no longer appears separate from the breast.

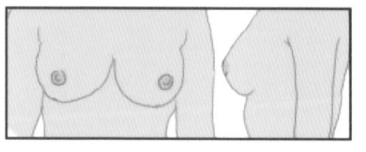

Sexual maturity in girls *(continued)*

Pubic hair development

Stage 1
No pubic hair is present.

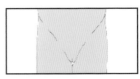

Stage 2
Straight hair begins to appear on the labia and extends between stages 2 and 3.

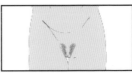

Stage 3
Pubic hair increases in quantity; it appears darker, curled, and more dense and begins to form the typical (but smaller in quantity) female triangle.

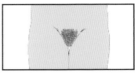

Stage 4
Pubic hair is more dense and curled; it's more adult in distribution, but less abundant than in an adult.

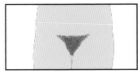

Stage 5
Pubic hair is abundant, appears in an adult female pattern, and may extend onto the medial part of the thighs.

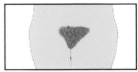

Minimizing the trauma of hospitalization

• Prepare a child for hospitalization and procedures to help the child cope more effectively and make it easier for him to trust the health care professionals responsible for his care.
• Consider the child's age, developmental stage, personality, and the length of the procedure or treatment when preparing him.
• Utilize child life specialists, who can explain procedures step by step and can also stay with the child during those procedures.
• Help the child and his family cope with fears associated with hospitalization by:
  – explaining procedures
  – answering questions openly and honestly
  – minimizing separation from the parents
  – structuring the environment to allow the child to retain as much control as possible.
• Foster family-centered care, which permits the family to remain as involved as possible and helps give the child and his family a sense of control in a difficult and unfamiliar situation.
• Use developmentally appropriate activities to help the child cope with the stress of hospitalization.

The importance of play

• Play is an excellent stress reducer and tension reliever. It allows the child freedom of expression to act out his fears, concerns, and anxieties.
• Play provides a source of diversion, alleviating separation anxiety.
• Play provides the child with a sense of safety and security because, while he's engaging in play, he knows that no painful procedures will occur.
• Developmentally appropriate play fosters the child's normal growth and development, especially for a child who's repeatedly hospitalized for a chronic condition.
• Play puts the child in the driver's seat, allowing him to make choices and giving him a sense of control.

Concepts of death in childhood

Developmental stage	Concept of death	Nursing considerations
Infancy	• None	• Be aware that the older infant will experience separation anxiety. • Help the family cope with death so they can be available to the infant.
Early childhood	• Knows the words "dead" and "death" • Reactions are influenced by the attitudes of his parents	• Help the family members (including siblings) cope with their feelings. • Allow the child to express his own feelings in an open and honest manner.
Middle childhood	• Understands universality and irreversibility of death • May have a fear of parents dying	• Use play to facilitate the child's understanding of death. • Allow siblings to express their feelings.
Late childhood	• Begins to incorporate family and cultural beliefs about death • Explores views of an afterlife • Faces the reality of own mortality	• Provide opportunities for the child to verbalize his fears. • Help the child discuss his concerns with his family.
Adolescence	• Has adult perception of death, but still focuses on the "here and now"	• Use opportunities to open discussion about death. • Allow expression of feelings of guilt, confusion, and anxiety. • Support and maintain the child's self-esteem.

Preparing children for surgery

What a child imagines about surgery is likely much more frightening than the reality. A child who knows what to expect ahead of time will be less fearful and more cooperative and will learn to trust his caregivers.

Before surgery

• Begin by asking the child to tell you what he thinks is going to happen during his surgery.
• Ask the child about worries or fears. Chances are, he'll be worried about something that isn't going to happen.
• Provide honest, age-appropriate explanations.
• Involve the parents (unless the adolescent would rather be prepared alone).
• Focus on what the child will see, hear, and feel; where his parents will be waiting for him; and when they'll be reunited.
• Encourage the child to ask questions.
• Reassure the child that he won't wake up during the surgery but that the doctor knows how and when to wake him up afterward.

• Show the child an induction mask (if it will be used) and allow him to "practice" by placing it on his face (or yours).
• Prepare the child for equipment (monitors, drains, and I.V. lines) he'll wake up with.
• Tell the child about the sights and sounds of the operating room.
• Tell the child that his doctor and nurse will be in the operating room with him. Reassure him that they'll talk to him and tell him what's happening.
• If possible, show the child where he'll be waking up in the recovery room and where his parents will be waiting for him.
• If the child will initially be cared for in an intensive care setting, allow him to visit the area ahead of time and to meet some of the nurses who will be caring for him.
• Tell the child it's perfectly fine to be afraid and to cry.
• After the surgery, encourage the child to talk about the experience; he may also express his feelings through art or play.

Preparing children for surgery (continued)

Many of the concerns that children have about hospitalization and surgery relate to their particular stage of development.

Age	Considerations
Infants, toddlers, and preschoolers	• Infants and toddlers are most concerned about separation from their parents, making separation during surgery especially difficult. • Because toddlers think concretely, showing is as important as telling when preparing toddlers for surgery. • Preschoolers may view medical procedures, including surgeries, as punishments for perceived bad behavior. • Preschoolers are also likely to have many misconceptions about what will happen during surgery.
School-age children	• School-age children have concerns about fitting in with peers and may view surgery as something that sets them apart from their friends. • A desire to appear "grown up" may make the school-age child reluctant to express his fears. • Despite a reluctance to express fear, school-age children are especially curious and interested in learning, are very receptive to preoperative teaching, and will likely ask many important questions (although they may need to be given "permission" to do so).
Adolescents	• Adolescents struggle with the conflict between wanting to assert their independence and needing their parents (and other adults) to take care of them during illness and treatment. • Adolescents may want to discuss their illness and treatment without a parent present. • In addition, adolescents may have a hard time admitting that they're afraid or experiencing pain or discomfort.

Child preventive care timeline for normal-risk children

Immunization**	Birth	1 mo	2 mo	3 mo	4 mo	5 mo	6 mo	12 mo	15 mo	18 mo	4 yr	6 yr	11 yr	12 yr	14 yr	16 yr	18 yr
Hepatitis B (HBV)*	Dose 1			Dose 2				Dose 3									
Polio (IPV)*			Dose 1		Dose 2				Dose 3		Dose 4						
Haemophilus influenzae type B (Hib)*			Dose 1		Dose 2		Dose 3		Dose 4								
Diphtheria, tetanus, pertussis (DTaP, Td)			Dose 1		Dose 2		Dose 3		Dose 4		Dose 5			Td once			
Measles, mumps, rubella (MMR)								Dose 1				Dose 2 OR	Dose 2				
Varicella (VZV)									Once								

Recommended by most U.S. authorities.

*Schedules may vary according to vaccine type.

**Note: For complete immunization information, see pages 71 to 73.

From *Child Health Guide: Put Prevention Into Practice*, U.S. Department of Health and Human Services, undated.

Age	Birth	1 yr	2 yr	3 yr	4 yr	5 yr	6 yr	7 yr	8 yr	9 yr	10 yr	11 yr	12 yr	13 yr	14 yr	15 yr	16 yr	17 yr	18 yr
Screening																			
Newborn screening: PKU, sickle cell, hypothyroidism	▓																		
Hearing	▓			▓															
Head circumference	Periodically																		
Height and weight	Periodically																		
Lead		▓																	
Eye screening				▓			Periodically												
Blood pressure					Periodically														
Dental health					▓		Periodically												
Alcohol use													Adolescents						
Counseling Development, nutrition, physical activity, safety, unintentional injuries and poisonings, violent behaviors and firearms, STDs and HIV, family planning, tobacco use, drug use	As appropriate for age																		

Birth history and early development

- Did the child's mother have a disease or another problem during the pregnancy?
- Was there birth trauma or a difficult delivery?
- Did the child arrive at developmental milestones—such as sitting up, walking, and talking—at the usual ages?
- Ask about childhood diseases and injuries and the presence of known congenital abnormalities.
- More specific questions will depend on which body system is being assessed.

Eyes and ears

- Look for clues to familial eye disorders, such as refractive errors and retinoblastoma (such as a family history of glaucoma).
- Does the child hold reading materials too close to his face while reading?
- Ask about behavior problems or poor performance in school.
- Ask about the child's birth history for risk of congenital hearing loss. (Maternal infection, maternal or infant use of ototoxic drugs, hypoxia, and trauma are all risk factors.)
- Ask the parents about behaviors that indicate possible hearing loss such as delayed speech development.

Respiratory system

- Ask the parents how often the child has upper respiratory tract infections.
- Find out if the child has had other respiratory signs and symptoms, such as a cough, dyspnea, wheezing, rhinorrhea, and a stuffy nose. Ask if these symptoms appear to be related to the child's activities or to seasonal changes.

Cardiovascular system

- Ask the parents if the child has difficulty keeping up physically with other children his age.
- Ask if the child experiences cyanosis on exertion, dyspnea, or orthopnea.
- Find out if the child assumes a squatting position or sleeps in the knee-chest position (either sign may indicate tetralogy of Fallot or another congenital heart defect).

GI system

- If the child has abdominal pain, ask him questions to help determine the pain's nature and severity.
- Determine the frequency and consistency of bowel movements and if the child suffers from constipation or diarrhea.

Pediatric health history (continued)

• Determine the characteristics of nausea and vomiting, especially projectile vomiting.

Urinary system

• Ask about a history of urinary tract malformations.
• Explore a history of discomfort with voiding and persistent enuresis after age 5.

Nervous system

• Find out if the child has experienced head or neck injuries, headaches, tremors, seizures, dizziness, fainting spells, or muscle weakness.
• Ask the parents if the child is overly active.

Musculoskeletal system

• Determine the ages at which the child reached major motor development milestones:
  – For an infant, these milestones include the age at which he held up his head, rolled over, sat unassisted, and walked alone.
  – For an older child, these milestones include the age at which the child first ran, jumped, walked up stairs, and pedaled a tricycle.
• Ask about a history of repeated fractures, muscle strains or sprains, painful joints, clumsiness, lack of coordination, abnormal gait, or restricted movement.

Hematologic and immune systems

• Check for anemia:
  – Ask the parents if the child has exhibited the common signs and symptoms of pallor, fatigue, failure to gain weight, malaise, and lethargy.
  – Ask the mother who's bottle-feeding if she uses an iron-fortified infant formula.
• Ask about the patient's history of infections. For an infant, 5 to 6 viral infections per year are normal; 8 to 12 are average for school-age children.
• Obtain a thorough history of allergic conditions.
• Ask about the family's history of infections and allergic or autoimmune disorders.

Endocrine system

• Obtain a thorough family history from one or both parents. Many endocrine disorders, such as diabetes mellitus and thyroid problems, can be hereditary. Others, such as delayed or precocious puberty, sometimes show a familial tendency.
• Ask about a history of poor weight gain, feeding problems, constipation, jaundice, hypothermia, or somnolence.

Age-specific interview and assessment tips

Infant

- Before performing a procedure, talk to and touch the infant.
- Use a gentle touch.
- Speak softly.
- Allow the infant to hold a favorite toy during the assessment.
- Let an older infant hold a small block in each hand.
- Remember that an older infant may be wary of strangers.
- Be alert to infant cues, such as crying, kicking, or waving arms.
- Perform traumatic procedures last when the infant is crying.
- Use distractions, such as bright objects, rattles, and talking.
- Enlist the parent's aid when examining the ears and mouth.
- Avoid abrupt, jerky movements.
- When the child is quiet, auscultate the heart, lungs, and abdomen.

Toddler

- Encourage the parents to be with you during the interview.
- Allow the toddler to be close to his parents.
- Provide simple explanations and use simple language.
- Use play as a communication tool.
- Tell the toddler that it's okay to cry.
- Watch for separation anxiety.

- Use the toddler's favorite toy as a tool during the interview. Encourage the toddler to use the toy for communication.
- Use play (count fingers or tickle toes) to assess body parts.
- Use parent assistance during the examination. For example, ask the parents to remove the toddler's outer clothing and help restrain the child during eye and ear examination.
- Use encouraging words during the examination.

Preschool child

- Ask simple questions.
- Allow the child to ask questions.
- Provide simple explanations.
- Avoid using words that sound threatening or have double meanings.
- Avoid slang words.
- Validate the child's perception.
- Use toys for expression.
- Use simple visual aids.
- Enlist the child's help during the examination, such as by allowing him to give you the stethoscope.
- Allow the child to touch and operate the diagnostic equipment.
- Explain what the child is going to feel before it happens. For example, explain that the stethoscope will be cold before using it on the child.

Age-specific interview and assessment tips
(continued)

• Utilize the child's imagination through puppets and play.
• Give the child choices when possible.

School-age child

• Provide explanations for procedures.
• Explain the purpose of equipment, such as an ophthalmoscope to see inside the eye.
• Avoid abstract explanations.
• Help the child vocalize his needs.
• Allow the child to engage in the conversation.
• Perform demonstration.
• Allow the child to undress himself.
• Respect the child's need for privacy.

Adolescent

• Give the adolescent control whenever possible.
• Facilitate trust and stress confidentiality.
• Encourage honest and open communication.
• Be nonjudgmental.
• Use clear explanations.
• Ask open-ended questions.
• Anticipate that the adolescent may be angry or upset.
• Ask if you can speak to the adolescent without the parent present.
• Ask the adolescent about parental involvement before initiating it.
• Give your undivided attention to the adolescent.
• Respect the adolescent's views, feeling, and differences.
• Allow the adolescent to undress in private, and provide the child with a gown.
• Expose only the area to be examined.
• Explain findings during the examination.
• Emphasize the normalcy of adolescent's development.
• Examine genitalia last but examine them as you would examine any other body part.

Normal heart rates in children

Age	Awake (beats/minute)	Asleep (beats/minute)	Exercise or fever (beats/minute)
Neonate	100 to 160	80 to 140	< 220
1 week to 3 months	100 to 220	80 to 200	< 220
3 months to 2 years	80 to 150	70 to 120	< 200
2 to 10 years	70 to 110	60 to 90	< 200
> 10 years	55 to 100	50 to 90	< 200

Normal blood pressure in children

Age	Weight (kg)	Systolic BP (mm Hg)	Diastolic BP (mm Hg)
Neonate	1	40 to 60	20 to 36
Neonate	2 to 3	50 to 70	30 to 45
1 month	4	64 to 96	30 to 62
6 months	7	60 to 118	50 to 70
1 year	10	66 to 126	41 to 91
2 to 3 years	12 to 14	74 to 124	39 to 89
4 to 5 years	16 to 18	79 to 119	45 to 85
6 to 8 years	20 to 26	80 to 124	45 to 85
10 to 12 years	32 to 42	85 to 135	55 to 88
>14 years	> 50	90 to 140	60 to 90

Normal respiratory rates in children

Age	Breaths per minute
Birth to 6 months	30 to 60
6 months to 2 years	20 to 30
3 to 10 years	20 to 28
10 to 18 years	12 to 20

Normal temperature ranges in children

Age	Temperature	
	° F	° C
Neonate	98.6 to 99.8	37 to 37.7
3 years	98.5 to 99.5	36.9 to 37.5
10 years	97.5 to 98.6	36.4 to 37
16 years	97.6 to 98.8	36.4 to 37.1

Measuring length

Because of an infant's tendency to be flexed and curled up, use these tips to help make assessing an infant's length easy and accurate:
• Place the infant's head in the midline position at the top of the measurement board.
• Hold one knee down with your hand and gently press it down toward the table until it's fully extended.
• Take the length measurement from the tip of the infant's head to his heel.

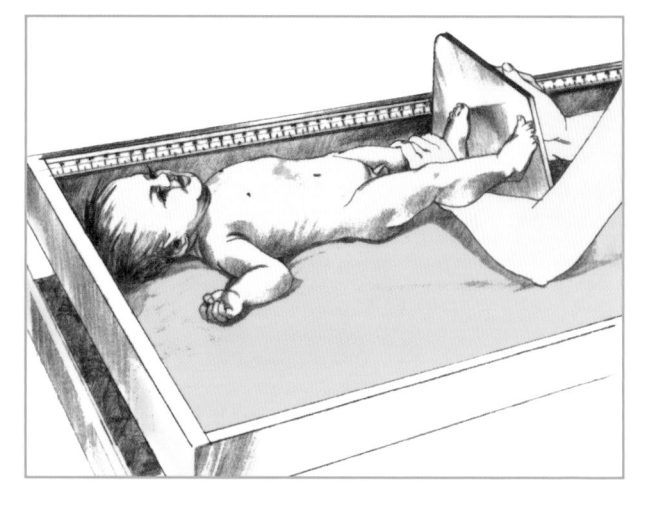

Measuring head circumference

To obtain an accurate head circumference measurement:
• Use a paper measuring tape to avoid stretching (as can happen with a cloth tape).
• Use landmarks—typically, place the tape just above the infant's eyebrows and around the occipital prominence at the back of the head to measure the largest diameter of the head.
• Take into consideration the shape of the infant's head and make adjustments as needed to measure the largest diameter.

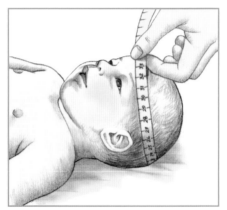

Cardiovascular assessment

Normal findings for a cardiovascular assessment are described below. Abnormal findings appear in color.

Inspection

• Skin is pink, warm, and dry.
• Chest is symmetrical.
• Pulsations may be visible in children with thin chest walls. The point of maximal impulse is commonly visible.
• Capillary refill is no more than 2 seconds.
• Cyanosis may be an early sign of a cardiac condition in an infant or a child.
• Dependent edema is a late sign of heart failure in children.

Palpation

• Pulses should be regular in rhythm and strength:
  – 4+ = bounding
  – 3+ = increased
  – 2+ = normal
  – 1+ = weak
  – 0 = absent
• No thrills or rubs are evident.

Auscultation

• Heart sounds are regular in rhythm, clear, and distinct (not weak or pounding, muffled, or distant).
• First heart sound (S_1) is heard best with stethoscope diaphragm over the mitral and tricuspid areas.
• Second heart sound (S_2) is heard best with stethoscope diaphragm over pulmonic and aortic areas.
• Third heart sound (S_3) is heard best with stethoscope bell over the mitral area. This sound is considered normal in some children and young adults but is abnormal when heard in older adults.
• S_4, if present, indicates the need for further cardiac evaluation because it's rarely heard as a normal heart sound.
• Murmurs in children may be innocent, functional, or organic. If a murmur is heard, note its location, timing within the cardiac cycle, intensity in relation to the child's position, and loudness.

Heart sound sites

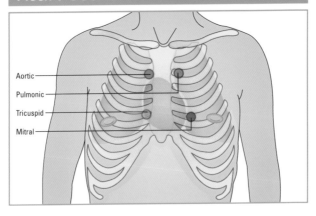

Aortic
Pulmonic
Tricuspid
Mitral

Grading murmurs

- **Grade I** is a barely audible murmur.
- **Grade II** is audible but quiet and soft.
- **Grade III** is moderately loud, without a thrust or thrill.
- **Grade IV** is loud, with a thrill.
- **Grade V** is very loud, with a palpable thrill.
- **Grade VI** is loud enough to be heard before the stethoscope comes into contact with the chest.

When recording your findings, use Roman numerals as part of a fraction, always with *VI* as the denominator. For instance, a grade III murmur would be recorded as *grade III/VI*.

Respiratory assessment

Normal findings for a respiratory assessment are described below. Abnormal findings appear in color.

Inspection

- Respirations are regular and effortless.
- No nasal flaring, grunting, or retractions are present.
- The presence of nasal flaring, expiratory grunting, and retractions are signs of respiratory distress in children.

Palpation

- Chest wall expands symmetrically on inspiration.
- Tactile fremitus is palpable.
- No rubs or vibrations are present.

Percussion

- Resonance is heard over most lung tissue.
- Dullness is normal over the heart area.

Auscultation

- Breath sounds normally sound louder and harsher than in adults due to the closeness of the stethoscope to the origins of the sound.
- Breath sounds are clear and equal; adventitious breath sounds are absent.
- Absent or diminished breath sounds are always abnormal and require further evaluation.

Looking for retractions

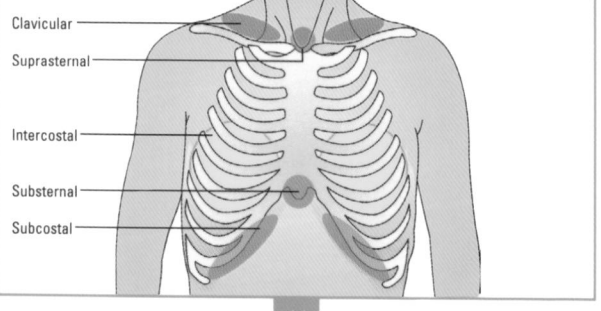

Clavicular
Suprasternal
Intercostal
Substernal
Subcostal

Qualities of normal breath sounds

Breath sound	Quality	Location
Tracheal	Harsh, high-pitched	Over trachea
Bronchial	Loud, high-pitched	Next to trachea
Bronchovesicular	Medium loudness and pitch	Next to sternum
Vesicular	Soft, low-pitched	Remainder of lungs

Abnormal breath sounds

Sound	Description
Crackles	Light crackling, popping, intermittent nonmusical sounds — like hairs being rubbed together — heard on inspiration or expiration
Pleural friction rub	Low-pitched, continual, superficial, squeaking or grating sound — like pieces of sandpaper being rubbed together — heard on inspiration and expiration
Rhonchi	Low-pitched, monophonic snoring sounds heard primarily on expiration but also throughout the respiratory cycle
Stridor	High-pitched, monophonic crowing sound heard on inspiration; louder in the neck than in the chest wall
Wheezes	High-pitched, continual musical or whistling sound heard primarily on expiration but sometimes also on inspiration

Pediatric coma scale

To quickly assess a patient's LOC and to uncover baseline changes, use the pediatric coma scale. This assessment tool grades consciousness in relation to eye opening and motor response and responses to auditory or visual stimuli. A decreased reaction score in one or more categories warns of an impending neurologic crisis. A patient scoring 7 or lower is comatose and probably has severe neurologic damage.

Test	Patient's reaction	Score
Best eye opening response	Open spontaneously	4
	Open to verbal command	3
	Open to pain	2
	No response	1
Best motor response	Obeys verbal command	6
	Localizes painful stimuli	5
	Flexion-withdrawal	4
	Flexion-abnormal (decorticate rigidity)	3
	Extension (decerebrate rigidity)	2
	No response	1
Best response to auditory and/or visual stimulus	*For a child older than age 2*	
	Oriented	5
	Confused	4
	Inappropriate words	3
	Incomprehensible sounds	2
	No response	1
	or	
	For a child younger than age 2	
	Smiles, listens, follows	5
	Cries, consolable	4
	Inappropriate persistent cry	3
	Agitated, restless	2
	No response	1

Total possible score: 3 to 15

Infant reflexes

Reflex	How to elicit	Age at disappearance
Trunk incurvature	When a finger is run laterally down the neonate's spine, the trunk flexes and the pelvis swings toward the stimulated side.	2 months
Tonic neck (fencing position)	When the neonate's head is turned while he's lying supine, the extremities on the same side extend outward while those on the opposite side flex.	2 to 3 months
Grasping	When a finger is placed in each of the neonate's hands, his fingers grasp tightly enough to be pulled to a sitting position.	3 to 4 months
Rooting	When the cheek is stroked, the neonate turns his head in the direction of the stroke.	3 to 4 months
Moro (startle reflex)	When lifted above the crib and suddenly lowered (or in response to a loud noise), the arms and legs symmetrically extend and then abduct while the fingers spread to form a "C."	4 to 6 months
Sucking	Sucking motion begins when a nipple is placed in the neonate's mouth.	6 months
Babinski's	When the sole on the side of the small toe is stroked, the neonate's toes fan upward.	2 years
Stepping	When held upright with the feet touching a flat surface, the neonate exhibits dancing or stepping movements.	Variable

Locating the fontanels

The locations of the anterior and posterior fontanels are depicted in this illustration of the top of a neonatal skull. The anterior fontanel typically closes by age 18 months, the posterior fontanel by age 2 months.

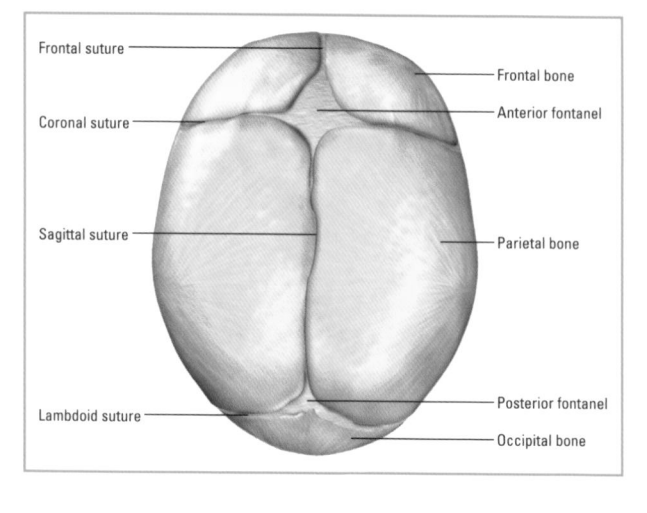

Frontal suture

Frontal bone

Coronal suture

Anterior fontanel

Sagittal suture

Parietal bone

Posterior fontanel

Lambdoid suture

Occipital bone

GI and GU assessment

Normal findings for a GI and GU assessment are described below. Abnormal findings appear in color.

Inspection

- GI: Abdomen symmetrical and fairly prominent when sitting or standing (flat when supine); no umbilical herniation
- GU: Urethra free from discharge or inflammation; no inguinal herniation; both testes descended
- Visible peristaltic waves may be a normal finding in infants and thin children; however, they may also indicate obstructive disorders such as pyloric stenosis.

Auscultation

- GI: Normal bowel sounds; possible borborygmi

- GU: No bruits over renal arteries
- Absent or hyperactive bowel sounds warrant further investigation because each usually indicates a GI disorder.

Percussion

- GI: Tympany over empty stomach or bowels; dullness over liver, full stomach, or stool in bowels
- GU: No tenderness or pain over kidneys

Palpation

- GI: No tenderness, masses, or pain; strong and equal femoral pulses
- GU: No tenderness or pain over kidneys

Tips for pediatric abdominal assessment

- Warm your hands before beginning the assessment.
- Note guarding of the abdomen and the child's ability to move around on the examination table.
- Flex the child's knees to decrease abdominal muscle tightening.
- Have the child use deep breathing or distraction during the examination; a parent can help divert the child's attention.
- Have the child "help" with the examination.
- Place your hand over the child's hand on the abdomen and extend your fingers beyond the child's fingers to decrease ticklishness when palpating the abdomen.
- Auscultate the abdomen before palpation (palpation can produce erratic bowel sounds); lightly palpate tender areas last.

Abdominal quadrants

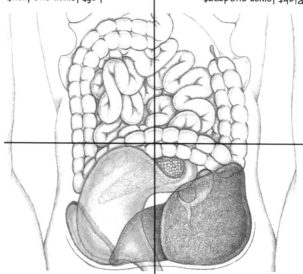

Right upper quadrant
- Right lobe of the liver
- Gallbladder
- Pylorus
- Duodenum
- Head of the pancreas
- Hepatic flexure of the colon
- Portions of the transverse and ascending colon

Left upper quadrant
- Left lobe of the liver
- Stomach
- Body of the pancreas
- Splenic flexure of the colon
- Portions of the transverse and descending colon

Right lower quadrant
- Cecum and appendix
- Portion of the ascending colon

Left lower quadrant
- Sigmoid colon
- Portion of the descending colon

50

Musculoskeletal assessment

Normal findings for a musculo-skeletal assessment are described below. Abnormal findings appear in color.

Inspection

- Extremities are symmetrical in length and size.
- No gross deformities are present.
- Good body alignment is evident.
- The child's gait is smooth with no involuntary movements.
- The child can perform active range of motion with no pain in all muscles and joints.

- No swelling or inflammation is present in joints or muscles.
- A lateral curvature of the spine indicates scoliosis.

Palpation

- Muscle mass shape is normal, with no swelling or tenderness.
- Muscles are equal in tone, texture, and shape bilaterally.
- No involuntary contractions or twitching is evident.
- Bilateral pulses are equally strong.

The 5 Ps of musculoskeletal injury

Pain

Ask the child whether he feels pain. If he does, assess its location, severity, and quality.

Paresthesia

Assess the child for loss of sensation by touching the injured area with the tip of an open safety pin. Abnormal sensation or loss of sensation indicates neurovascular involvement.

Paralysis

Assess whether the patient can move the affected area. If he

can't, he might have nerve or tendon damage.

Pallor

Paleness, discoloration, and coolness on the injured side may indicate neurovascular compromise.

Pulse

Check all pulses distal to the injury site. If a pulse is decreased or absent, blood supply to the area is reduced.

Sequence of tooth eruption

A child's primary and secondary teeth will erupt in a predictable order, as shown in these illustrations.

Primary tooth eruption

Maxilla (upper teeth)

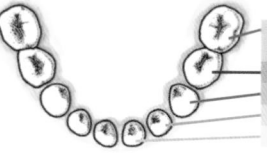

Teeth	Age of eruption
Central incisors	8 to 12 months
Lateral incisors	9 to 13 months
Canines	16 to 22 months
First molars	Boys: 13 to 19 months Girls: 14 to 18 months
Second molars	25 to 33 months

Second molars	Boys: 23 to 31 months Girls: 24 to 30 months
First molars	14 to 18 months
Canines	17 to 23 months
Lateral incisors	10 to 16 months
Central incisors	6 to 10 months

Mandible (lower teeth)

Sequence of tooth eruption (continued)

Secondary (or permanent) tooth eruption

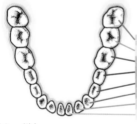

Maxilla (upper teeth)

Teeth	Age of eruption
Central incisors	7 to 8 years
Lateral incisors	8 to 9 years
Cuspids	11 to 12 years
First bicuspids	10 to 11 years
Second bicuspids	10 to 12 years
First molars	6 to 7 years
Second molars	12 to 13 years
Third molars	Variable

Teeth	Age of eruption
Third molars	17 to 21 years
Second molars	11 to 13 years
First molars	6 to 7 years
Second bicuspids	11 to 12 years
First bicuspids	10 to 12 years
Cuspids	9 to 10 years
Lateral incisors	7 to 8 years
Central incisors	6 to 7 years

Mandible (lower teeth)

Pain assessment

Assessing pain in infants and young children requires the cooperation of the parents and the use of age-specific assessment tools. If the child can communicate verbally, he can also aid in the process.

History questions

To help you better understand the child's pain, ask the parents these questions:
• What kinds of pain has your child had in the past?
• How does your child usually respond to pain?
• How do you know your child is in pain?
• What do you do when he's hurting?
• What does your child do when he's hurting?
• What works best to relieve your child's pain?
• Is there anything special you would like me to know about your child and pain?

Behavioral responses to pain

Behavior is the language infants and children rely on to convey information about their pain. In an infant, facial expression is the most common and consistent behavioral response to all stimuli, painful or pleasurable, and may be the single best indicator of pain for the provider and the parent. Facial expressions that tend to indicate that the infant is in pain include:
• mouth stretched open
• eyes tightly shut
• brows and forehead knitted (as they are in a grimace)
• cheeks raised high enough to form a wrinkle on the nose.

In young children, facial expression is joined by other behaviors to convey pain. In these patients, look for such signs as:
• narrowing of the eyes
• grimace or fearful appearance
• frequent and longer-lasting bouts of crying, with a tone that's higher and louder than normal
• less receptiveness to comforting by parents or other caregivers
• holding or protecting the painful area.

FLACC Scale

The Face, Legs, Activity, Cry, Consolability (FLACC) Scale uses the characteristics listed below to measure pain in infants.

The FLACC is a behavioral pain assessment scale for use in nonverbal patients unable to provide reports of pain. Here's how to use it: 1. Rate patient in each of the five measurement categories; 2. Add scores together; 3. Document total pain score.

Category	Score		
	0	1	2
Face	No particular expression or smile	Occasional grimace or frown, withdrawn, disinterested	Frequent to constant frown, clenched jaw, and quivering chin
Legs	Normal position or relaxed	Uneasy, restless, tense	Kicking or legs drawn up
Activity	Lying quietly, normal position, moves easily	Squirming, shifting back/forth, tense	Arched, rigid, or jerking
Cry	No cry (awake or asleep)	Moans or whimpers, occasional complaint	Crying steadily, screams or sobs, frequent complaints
Consolability	Content, relaxed	Reassured by occasional touching, hugging, or "talking to," distractible	Difficult to console or comfort

Adapted with permission from "The FLACC: A behavioral scale for scoring postoperative pain in young children," by S. Merkel, et al. *Pediatric Nursing,* 23(3), 1997, p. 293-297.

Measuring pain in young children

For children who are old enough to speak and understand sufficiently, three useful tools can help them communicate information for measuring their pain. Here's how to use each one.

Visual analog scale

A visual analog pain scale is simply a straight line with the phrase "no pain" at one end and the phrase "the most pain possible" at the other. Children who understand the concept of a continuum can mark the spot on the line that corresponds to the level of pain they feel.

| No pain |————————————————————| The most pain possible |

Wong-Baker FACES Pain Rating Scale

The child age 3 and older can use the faces scale to rate his pain. When using this tool, make sure he can see and point to each face and then describe the amount of pain each face is experiencing. If he's able, the child can read the text under the picture; otherwise, you or his parent can read it to him.

Avoid saying anything that might prompt the child to choose a certain face. Then ask the child to choose the face that shows how he's feeling right now. Record his response in your assessment notes.

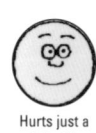
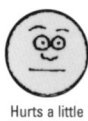
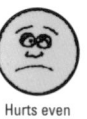

| Happy because he doesn't hurt at all | Hurts just a little bit | Hurts a little more | Hurts even more | Hurts a whole lot | Hurts the most |

Reprinted with permission from Wong, D.L., et al. *Wong's Essentials of Pediatric Nursing*, 6th ed. St. Louis: Mosby–Year Book, Inc., 2001.

Measuring pain in young children *(continued)*

Chip tool

The chip tool uses four identical chips to signify levels of pain and can be used for the child who understands the basic concept of adding one thing to another to get more. If available, you can use poker chips. If not, simply cut four uniform circles from a sheet of paper. Here's how to present the chips:

• First say, "I want to talk with you about the hurt you might be having right now."

• Next, align the chips horizontally on the bedside table, a clipboard, or other firm surface where the child can easily see and reach them.

• Point to the chip at the child's far left and say, "This chip is just a little bit of hurt."

• Point to the second chip and say, "This next chip is a little more hurt."

• Point to the third chip and say, "This next chip is a lot of hurt."

• Point to the last chip and say, "This last chip is the most hurt you can have."

• Ask the child, "How many pieces of hurt do you have right now?" (You won't need to offer the option of "no hurt at all" because the child will tell you if he doesn't hurt.)

• Record the number of chips. If the child's answer isn't clear, talk to him about his answer, and then record your findings.

Common pediatric pain medications

Drug	Considerations
Opioids	
Morphine	• Give single I.V. doses slowly over at least 5 minutes. • Use only preservative-free preparations in neonates. • Monitor the patient for respiratory depression after administration.
Fentanyl	• Infuse I.V. doses slowly, over at least 5 minutes. • Instruct the child to suck on lozenges, not chew them. • Monitor the patient for respiratory depression after administration.
Hydromorphone	• Monitor the patient for respiratory depression after administration. • Assess for pain relief 30 minutes after administration.
Nonopioids	
Acetaminophen	• Watch for signs and symptoms of hepatotoxicity after administration, even with moderate doses. • Don't administer more than 5 doses in 24 hours.
Ibuprofen	• Instruct the patient (or his parents) that the drug should be taken with meals or milk to reduce the risk of GI upset. • Tablets may be crushed if the child can't swallow them; other alternatives include using suspension or drops.
Naproxen	• Use suspension if the child can't swallow tablets. • Give the drug with food to reduce the risk of GI upset.

Causes of burns

Type	Causes
Thermal	Flames, radiation, or excessive heat from fire, steam, or hot liquids or objects
Chemical	Various acids, bases, and caustics
Electrical	Electrical current and lightning
Light	Intense light sources or ultraviolet light, including sunlight
Radiation	Nuclear radiation and ultraviolet light

Classifying burns

Burns are classified according to the depth of the injury, as follows:
• **First-degree burns** are limited to the epidermis. Sunburn is a typical first-degree burn. These burns are painful but self-limiting. They don't lead to scarring and require only local wound care.
• **Second-degree burns** extend into the dermis but leave some residual dermis viable. These burns are painful and the skin will appear swollen and red with blister formation.
• **Third-degree,** or **full-thickness, burns** involve the destruction of the entire dermis, leaving only subcutaneous tissue exposed. These burns look dry and leathery and are painless because the nerve endings are destroyed.
• **Fourth-degree burns** are a rare type of burn usually associated with lethal injury. They extend beyond the subcutaneous tissue, involving the muscle, fasciae, and bone. Occasionally termed *transmural burns,* these injuries are commonly associated with complete transection of an extremity.

Estimating the extent of burns

Lund-Browder chart

Use to estimate the extent of an infant's or a child's (up to age 7) burns.

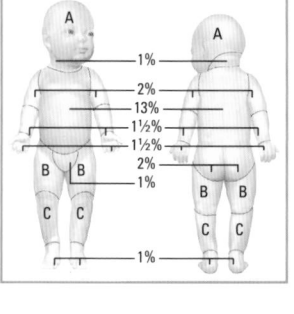

Rule of Nines

Use to estimate the extent of an older child's or a teenager's burns.

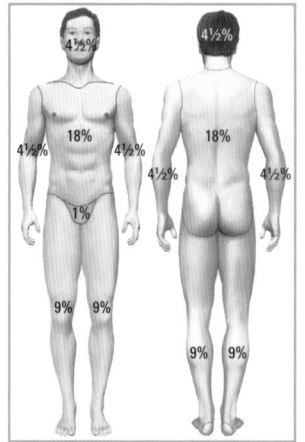

Relative percentages of areas affected by age

At birth	0 to 1 yr	1 to 4 yr	5 to 9 yr	10 to 15 yr	16+ yr
A: Half of head					
9½%	8½%	6½%	5½%	4½%	3½%
B: Half of thigh					
2½%	3½%	4%	4½%	4½%	4½%
C: Half of leg					
2½%	2½%	2½%	3%	3½%	3½%

Recognizing child abuse and neglect

If you suspect a child is being harmed, contact your local child protective services or the police. Contact the Childhelp USA National Child Abuse Hotline (1-800-4-A-CHILD) to find out where and how to file a report.

The following signs may indicate child abuse or neglect.

Children

- Show sudden changes in behavior or school performance
- Haven't received help for physical or medical problems brought to the parent's attention
- Are always watchful, as if preparing for something bad to happen
- Lack adult supervision
- Are overly compliant, passive, or withdrawn
- Come to school or activities early, stay late, and don't want to go home

Parents

- Show little concern for the child
- Deny or blame the child for the child's problems in school or at home
- Request that teachers or caregivers use harsh physical discipline if the child misbehaves
- See the child as entirely bad, worthless, or burdensome
- Demand a level of physical or academic performance the child can't achieve
- Look primarily to the child for care, attention, and satisfaction of emotional needs

Parents and children

- Rarely look at each other
- Consider their relationship to be entirely negative
- State that they don't like each other

Signs of child abuse

Here are some signs associated with specific types of child abuse and neglect. These types of abuse are typically found in combination rather than alone.

Physical abuse

• Has unexplained burns, bites, bruises, broken bones, black eyes
• Has fading bruises or marks after absence from school
• Cries when it's time to go home
• Shows fear at approach of adults
• Reports injury by parent or caregiver

Neglect

• Is frequently absent from school
• Begs or steals food or money
• Lacks needed medical or dental care, immunizations, or glasses
• Is consistently dirty and has severe body odor
• Lacks sufficient clothing for the weather

Sexual abuse

• Has difficulty walking or sitting
• Suddenly refuses to change for gym or join in physical activities
• Reports nightmares or bedwetting
• Demonstrates bizarre, sophisticated, or unusual sexual knowledge or behavior
• Becomes pregnant or contracts a venereal disease when younger than age 14

Emotional maltreatment

• Shows extremes in behavior, such as overly compliant or demanding behavior, extreme passivity, or aggression
• Is inappropriately adult (parenting other children) or inappropriately infantile (frequent rocking or head banging)
• Shows delayed physical or emotional development
• Reports a lack of attachment to the parent
• Has attempted suicide

Suicide warning signs

Watch for these warning signs of impending suicide:
• withdrawal or social isolation
• signs of depression, which may include crying, fatigue, helplessness, hopelessness, poor concentration, reduced interest in daily activities, sadness, constipation, and weight loss
• farewells to friends and family
• putting affairs in order
• giving away prized possessions
• expression of covert suicide messages and death wishes
• obvious suicide messages such as, "I would be better off dead."

Answering a threat

If a patient shows signs of impending suicide, assess the seriousness of the intent and the immediacy of the risk. Consider a patient with a chosen method who plans to commit suicide in the next 48 to 72 hours a high risk.

Tell the patient that you're concerned. Urge him to avoid self-destructive behavior until the staff has an opportunity to help him. Consult with the treatment team about psychiatric hospitalization.

Initiate the following safety precautions for those at high risk for suicide:
• Provide a safe environment.
• Remove dangerous objects, such as belts, razors, suspenders, electric cords, glass, knives, nail files, and clippers.
• Make the patient's specific restrictions clear to staff members, and plan for observation of the patient.
• Stay alert when the patient is shaving, taking medication, or using the bathroom.
• Encourage continuity of care and consistency of primary nurses.

Notes

Comprehensive metabolic panel

Test	Conventional units	SI units
Albumin	3.5 to 5 g/dl	35 to 50 g/L
Alkaline phosphatase	2 to 10 yr: 100 to 300 units/L 11 to 18 yr: Male: 50 to 375 units/L; Female: 30 to 300 units/L	2 to 10 yr: 100 to 300 units/L 11 to 18 yr: Male: 50 to 375 units/L; Female: 30 to 300 units/L
ALT	< 1 yr: 5 to 28 units/L > 1 yr: 820 units/L	< 1 yr: 5 to 28 units/L > 1 yr: 820 units/L
AST	< 1 yr: 15 to 60 units/L > 1 yr: ≤ 20 units/L	< 1 yr: 15 to 60 units/L > 1 yr: ≤ 20 units/L
Bilirubin, total	< 10 mg/dl	< 171 µmol/L
BUN	5 to 20 mg/dl	2 to 7 mmol/L
Calcium, ionized	4.48 to 4.92 mg/dl	1.12 to 1.23 mmol/L
Calcium, total	8 to 10.5 mg/dl	2 to 2.6 mmol/L
Carbon dioxide	22 to 26 mEq/L	22 to 26 mmol/L
Chloride	94 to 106 mEq/L	94 to 106 mmol/L
Creatinine	0.3 to 0.7 mg/dl	27 to 62 µmol/L
Glucose	60 to 105 mg/dl	3.3 to 5.8 mmol/L
Potassium	3.5 to 5 mEq/L	3.5 to 5 mmol/L
Protein, total	6.5 to 8.6 g/dl	65 to 86 g/L
Sodium	135 to 145 mEq/L	135 to 145 mmol/L

Thyroid panel

Test	Conventional units	SI units
Triiodothyronine (T₃)	1 to 5 yr: 105 to 269 ng/dl 5 to 10 yr: 94 to 241 ng/dl 10 to 15 yr: 83 to 215 ng/dl	1 to 5 yr: 1.62 to 4.14 nmol/L 5 to 10 yr: 1.45 to 3.71 nmol/L 10 to 15 yr: 1.28 to 3.31 nmol/L
Thyroxine (T₄), free	0.7 to 1.7 ng/dl	9 to 22 pmol/L
T₄, total	1 to 5 yr: 7.3 to 15 mcg/dl 5 to 10 yr: 6.4 to 13.3 mcg/dl 10 to 15 yr: 5.6 to 11.7 mcg/dl	1 to 5 yr: 94 to 194 nmol/L 5 to 10 yr: 83 to 172 nmol/L 10 to 15 yr: 72 to 151 nmol/L
TSH	0.4 to 4.2 µunits/L	0 to 5.5 mIU/ml

Other chemistry tests

Test	Conventional units	SI units
Ammonia	13 to 48 mcg/dl	9 to 34 µmol/L
Amylase	>1 yr: 26 to 102 units/L	>1 yr: 26 to 102 units/L
Anion gap	7 to 14 mEq/L	7 to 14 mmol/L
Bilirubin, direct	<0.5 mg/dl	<6.8 µmol/L
Calcium, ionized	4.48 to 4.92 mg/dl	1.12 to 1.23 mmol/L
Cortisol	a.m.: 8 to 18 mcg/dl	225 to 505 nmol/L
	p.m.: 16 to 36 mcg/dl	450 to 1010 nmol/L
C-reactive protein	<0.8 mg/dl	<8 mg/L
Ferritin	7 to 144 ng/ml	7 to 144 mcg/L
Folate	1.8 to 9.0 ng/ml	4 to 20 nmol/L
GGT	0 to 23 units/L	0 to 23 units/L
Glycosylated hemoglobin (HbA₁c)	3.9% to 7.7%	0.039 to 0.077
Iron	53 to 119 mcg/dl	9.5 to 27 µmol/L
Iron-binding capacity	250 to 400 mcg/dl	45 to 72 µmol/L
Magnesium	1.5 to 2.0 mEq/l	0.75 to 1 mmol/L
Osmolality	285 to 295 mOsm/kg	285 to 295 mOsm/kg
Phosphate	1 yr: 3.8 to 6.2 mg/dl	1 yr: 1.23 to 2 mmol/L
	2 to 5 yr: 3.5 to 6.8 mg/dl	2 to 5 yr: 1.03 to 2.2 mmol/L
Uric acid	2 to 7 mg/dl	120 to 420 µmol/L

Complete blood count with differential

Test	Conventional units	SI units
Hemoglobin	2 to 6 mo: 10.7 to 17.3 g/dl	2 to 6 mo: 107 to 173 mmol/L
	1 to 12 yr: 9.5 to 14.1 g/dl	1 to 12 yr: 95 to 141 mmol/L
	6 to 16 yr: 10.3 to 14.9 g/dl	6 to 16 yr: 103 to 149 mmol/L
Hematocrit	2 to 6 mo: 35% to 49%	2 to 6 mo: 0.35 to 0.49
	6 mo to 1 yr: 29% to 43%	6 mo to 1 yr: 0.29 to 0.43
	1 to 6 yr: 30% to 40%	1 to 6 yr: 0.30 to 0.40
	6 to 16 yr: 32% to 42%	6 to 16 yr: 0.32 to 0.42
RBC	6 mo to 1 yr: 3.8 to $5.2 \times 10^6/mm^3$	6 mo. to 1 yr: 3.8 to $5.2 \times 10^{12}/L$
	6 to 16 yr: 4 to $5.2 \times 10^6/mm^3$	6 to 16 yr: 4 to $5.2 \times 10^{12}/L$
MCH	2 to 6 yr: 24 to 30 pg/cell	2 to 6 yr: 0.37 to 0.47 fmol/cell
	6 to 12 yr: 25 to 33 pg/cell	6 to 12 yr: 0.39 to 0.51 fmol/cell
	12 to 18 yr: 25 to 35 pg/cell	12 to 18 yr: 0.39 to 0.53 fmol/cell
MCHC	34 g/dl	340 g/L
MCV	2 to 6 yr: 82 mm^3	2 to 6 yr: 82 fL
	6 to 12 yr: 86 mm^3	6 to 12 yr: 86 fL
	12 to 18 yr: 88 mm^3	12 to 18 yr: 88 fL
WBC	2 mo to 6 yr: 5,000 to 19,000 cells/mm^3	2 mo to 6 yr: 5 to 19×10^9
	6 to 18 yr: 4,800 to 10,800 cells/mm^3	6 to 18 yr: 4.8 to 10.8×10^9
Bands	5% to 11%	0.05 to 0.11
Basophils	0%	0
Eosinophils	0% to 3%	0 to 0.03
Lymphocytes	25% to 76%	0.25 to 0.76
Monocytes	0% to 5%	0 to 0.05
Neutrophils	54% to 62%	0.54 to 0.62
Platelets	150,000 to 450,000/mm^3	150 to $450 \times 10^9/L$

Antibiotic peaks and troughs

Test		Conventional units	SI units
Amikacin	Peak	20 to 30 mcg/ml	34 to 52 µmol/L
	Trough	1 to 4 mcg/ml	2 to 7 µmol/L
Chloramphenicol	Peak	15 to 25 mcg/ml	46.4 to 77 µmol/L
	Trough	5 to 15 mcg/ml	15.5 to 46.4 µmol/L
Gentamicin	Peak	4 to 8 mcg/ml	4 to 16.7 µmol/L
	Trough	1 to 2 mcg/ml	2.1 to 4.2 µmol/L
Tobramycin	Peak	4 to 8 mcg/ml	4 to 16.7 µmol/L
	Trough	1 to 2 mcg/ml	2.1 to 4.2 µmol/L
Vancomycin	Peak	25 to 40 mcg/ml	17 to 27 µmol/L
	Trough	5 to 10 mcg/ml	3.4 to 6.8 µmol/L

Urine tests

Test	Conventional units	SI units
Urinalysis		
Appearance	Clear to slightly hazy	—
Color	Straw to dark yellow	—
pH	4.5 to 8	—
Specific gravity	1.005 to 1.035	—
Glucose	None	—
Protein	None	—
RBCs	None or rare	—
WBCs	None or rare	—
Osmolality	50 to 1,200 mOsm/kg	—

Lipid panel (children ages 2 to 19)

Test	Conventional units	SI units
Total cholesterol	Acceptable: < 170 mg/dl; Borderline: 170 to 199 mg/dl; High: $\geq$ 200 mg/dl	—
LDL	Acceptable: < 110 mg/dl; Borderline: 110 to 129 mg/dl; High: $\geq$ 130 mg/dl	—
HDL	$\geq$ 35 mg/dl	—
Triglycerides	$\leq$ 150 mg/dl	—

Recognizing acid-base disorders

Disorder	ABG findings	Possible causes
Respiratory acidosis (excess CO_2 retention)	• pH < 7.35 • HCO_3^- > 26 mEq/L (if compensating) • $Paco_2$ > 45 mm Hg	• Central nervous system depression from drugs, injury, or disease • Hypoventilation from respiratory, cardiac, musculoskeletal, or neuromuscular disease
Respiratory alkalosis (excess CO_2 loss)	• pH > 7.45 • HCO_3^- < 22 mEq/L (if compensating) • $Paco_2$ < 35 mm Hg	• Hyperventilation due to anxiety, pain, or improper ventilator settings • Respiratory stimulation from drugs, disease, hypoxia, fever, or high room temperature • Gram-negative bacteremia
Metabolic acidosis (HCO_3^- loss or acid retention)	• pH < 7.35 • HCO_3^- < 22 mEq/L • $Paco_2$ < 35 mm Hg (if compensating)	• Depletion of HCO_3^- from renal disease, diarrhea, or small-bowel fistulas • Excessive production of organic acids from hepatic disease, endocrine disorders such as diabetes mellitus, hypoxia, shock, or drug toxicity • Inadequate excretion of acids due to renal disease
Metabolic alkalosis (HCO_3^- retention or acid loss)	• pH > 7.45 • HCO_3^- > 26 mEq/L • $Paco_2$ > 45 mm Hg (if compensating)	• Loss of hydrochloric acid from prolonged vomiting or gastric suctioning • Loss of potassium from increased renal excretion (as in diuretic therapy) or corticosteroid overdose • Excessive alkali ingestion

Childhood immunization schedule

Recommended immunization schedule for persons aged 0–6 years—United States, 2007

Vaccine / Age	Birth	1 mo	2 mo	4 mo	6 mo	12 mo	15 mo	18 mo	19-23 mo	2-3 yr	4-6 yr
Hepatitis B	HepB	HepB			HepB						HepB series
Rotavirus			Rota	Rota	Rota						
Diphtheria, tetanus, pertussis			DTaP	DTaP	DTaP		DTaP				DTaP
Haemophilus influenzae type b			Hib	Hib	Hib	Hib			Hib		
Pneumococcal			PCV	PCV	PCV	PCV				PCV PPV	
Inactivated poliovirus			IPV	IPV	IPV					IPV	IPV
Influenza					Influenza (yearly)						
Measles, mumps, rubella						MMR					MMR
Varicella						Varicella					Varicella
Hepatitis A						HepA (2 doses)				HepA series	
Meningococcal										MPSV4	

Key:
■ Range of recommended ages ■ Catch-up immunization ■ Certain high-risk groups

For more detailed information, see Centers for Disease Control and Prevention. Recommended immunization schedules for persons aged 0–18 years—United States, 2007. MMWR 2006;55(51&52):Q1–Q4.

Meds/IV

Catch-up immunization schedule

Recommended immunization schedule for persons aged 7–18 years—United States, 2007

Vaccine	Age	7–10 years	11–12 years	13–14 years	15 years	16–18 years
Tetanus, diphtheria, pertussis		See full schedule	Tdap		Tdap	
Human papillomavirus		See full schedule	HPV (3 doses)		HPV series	
Meningococcal		MPSV4	MCV4		MCV4 / MCV4	
Pneumococcal			PPV			
Influenza			Influenza (yearly)			
Hepatitis A			HepA series			
Hepatitis B			HepB series			
Inactivated poliovirus			IPV series			
Measles, mumps, rubella			MMR series			
Varicella			Varicella series			

Key: ▢ Range of recommended ages   ▢ Catch-up immunization   ▢ Certain high-risk groups

For more detailed informations, see Centers for Disease Control and Prevention. Recommended immunization schedules for persons aged 0–18 years—United States, 2007. MMWR 2006;55(51&52):Q1–Q4.

Meds/IV

Catch-up immunizations

Protection from certain serious communicable diseases can be obtained through immunization with a variety of vaccines. Without proper immunization, these diseases can cause chronic illness, disability, cancer, or death. Most immunizations are given in a series during infancy and childhood and provide lifelong protection if the series is completed. Some vaccines, such as tetanus, require booster shots to maintain immunity.

If a child hasn't had access to medical care, has been seriously ill, or is an immigrant, he might not have received the recommended immunizations. Catch-up immunizations should be administered to protect that child and to protect others from exposure in such facilities as daycares and schools.

Complete information about catch-up immunizations can be found at *www.cdc.gov/nip/recs/child-schedule.htm.*

Dosage calculation formulas and common conversions

Common calculations

$$\text{child's dose in mg} = \text{child's BSA in m}^2 \times \frac{\text{pediatric dose in mg}}{\text{m}^2/\text{day}}$$

$$\text{child's dose in mg} = \frac{\text{child's BSA in m}^2}{\text{average adult BSA (1.73 m}^2)} \times \text{average adult dose}$$

$$\text{mcg/ml} = \text{mg/ml} \times 1{,}000$$

$$\text{ml/minute} = \frac{\text{ml/hour}}{60}$$

$$\text{mg/minute} = \frac{\text{mg in bag}}{\text{ml in bag}} \times \text{flow rate} \div 60$$

$$\text{mcg/minute} = \frac{\text{mg in bag}}{\text{ml in bag}} \div 0.06 \times \text{flow rate}$$

$$\text{mcg/kg/minute} = \frac{\text{mcg/ml} \times \text{ml/minute}}{\text{weight in kg}}$$

Common conversions

1 kg = 1,000 g	1 L = 1,000 ml	8 oz = 240 ml
1 g = 1,000 mg	1 ml = 1,000 microliters	1 oz = 30 g
1 mg = 1,000 mcg	1 tsp = 5 ml	1 lb = 454 g
	1 tbs = 15 ml	2.2 lb = 1 kg
1" = 2.54 cm	2 tbs = 30 ml	

Estimating BSA in children

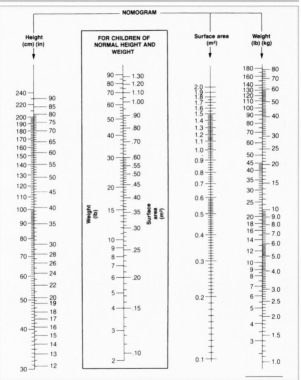

Adapted with permission from Behrman, R.E., et al. *Nelson Textbook of Pediatrics,* 16th ed. Philadelphia: W.B. Saunders Co., 2000.

Meds/IV

I.M. injection sites in children

When selecting the best site for a child's I.M. injection, consider the child's age, weight, and muscle development; the amount of subcutaneous fat over the injection site; the type of drug you're administering; and the drug's absorption rate. These guidelines may assist you in making a selection.

Vastus lateralis

• The rectus femoris muscle should be avoided when using this injection site.

Appropriate age
• Infants
• Toddlers

Needle size and length
• Infants under 4 months: 23 to 25 gauge, ⅝"
• Infants over 4 months and toddlers: 22 to 25 gauge, 1"

Recommended maximum amount
• Give 1 ml or less to infants.
• Give 2 ml or less to toddlers.

Special considerations
• The vastus lateralis is a large, well-developed muscle with few major blood vessels or nerves.

Ventrogluteal

Appropriate age
• Infants
• Toddlers
• Preschool and older children
• Adolescents

Needle size and length
• 23 to 25 gauge, ⅝" needle for infants less than 4 months
• 22 to 25 gauge, 1" needle for all other age-groups

Recommended maximum amount
• Give 1 ml or less to infants.
• Give 2 ml or less to toddlers.
• Give 3 ml or less to preschool and older children.
• Give 5 ml or less to adolescents.

Special considerations
• This site is less painful than the vastus lateralis.
• This site is also relatively free from major nerves and blood vessels.

Dorsogluteal

Appropriate age
• Children older than age 2 years

Needle size and length
• 20 to 25 gauge, 1/2" to 1 1/2" needle

Recommended maximum amount
• Give 1.5 ml or less to children ages 2 to 6
• Give 2 ml or less to children over age 6

Special considerations
• This site isn't recommended for children who haven't been walking for at least a year.
• Injury to the sciatic nerve is possible when using this site.

- Posterior superior iliac crest
- Greater trochanter
- Injection site
- Sciatic nerve

Deltoid

Appropriate age
• Toddlers
• Preschool and older children
• Adolescents

Needle size and length
• 22 to 25 gauge, 5/8" to 1" needle in all age-groups

Recommended maximum amount
• Give 1 ml or less in toddlers and preschool and older children
• Give 1 to 1 1/2 ml in adolescents

Special considerations
• This site is associated with less pain than the vastus lateralis site.
• Because blood flows faster in the deltoid muscle than in other muscle sites, drug absorption is faster.
• Injury to the radial nerve is possible when using this site.

- Brachial artery
- Radial nerve
- Injection site

Tips for pediatric injections

When giving a child an injection, the major goal should be to minimize trauma and discomfort while providing safe, efficient administration of a necessary medicine or vaccination.

To most toddlers and preschoolers—and to many older children—
the prospect of an injection is the most frightening part of a doctor's
visit or even a hospitalization. Many strategies, including those outlined here, can be used to minimize the trauma of receiving an injection, while establishing trust between the child and the health care
team and making future injections easier for the child (and for the
nurse who's giving the injection).

Medicine to keep you healthy

• Give the child a simple, age-appropriate explanation for why the
injection is being given. When a child is being vaccinated, that explanation might be, "This shot will give you medicine to keep you from
getting sick." (Young children may think an injection is being given as
a punishment and may not even realize that medication is being
given.)
• Allow the child to give a "shot" to a doll or stuffed animal to give
him a sense of control, to let him see that the injection has a beginning and an end, and to give him a clear understanding of what will
happen.

The best policy

• Be honest; tell the child that it will hurt for a moment but that it will
be over quickly. (Honesty promotes trust; if a nurse is honest about
the potential for pain, the child will believe her when she tells him
something won't hurt.)

Coping and comfort

• Give the child a coping strategy, such as squeezing his mother's
hand, counting to five, singing a song, and looking away.
• Have a parent hold and comfort the child while the injection is being
given. A parent's presence reassures the child that nothing truly bad
will happen. (The child may actually cry more when a parent is present, but this is because he feels safe enough to do so.)

Tips for pediatric injections *(continued)*

Praise and cover

• When the injection has been given, tell the child that "the hurting part" is over, and praise him for what a good job he did (regardless of how he reacted). Never tell a child to "be brave," to "be a big boy," or not to cry, as these requests will set the child up for failure.
• Give the child a bandage. (A young child may not believe the "hurting part" is over until a bandage has been applied.)
• Always give injections in a designated treatment area. Avoid performing painful procedures in a playroom or, if possible, in the child's hospital room, because he needs to know there are places where he can feel completely safe.

Giving the injection

• Apply firm pressure at the site for 10 to 15 seconds immediately before giving the injection to decrease discomfort (a numbing patch may be used).
• When two or more injections are needed, give them simultaneously in different extremities; have two or more nurses assist (and provide manual restraint, if needed) during the procedures. (The child has only one painful experience when multiple injections are given simultaneously; this is believed to be less traumatic than receiving painful injections one after the other.)
• Apply bandages to each site, and immediately comfort and console the child following the injections.
• Always keep resuscitation equipment and epinephrine readily available in case of an anaphylactic response to an immunization.

Performing intraosseous administration

In an emergency, intraosseous drug administration may be used for a critically ill child younger than age 6. Insert a bone marrow needle (or spinal needle with stylette, trephine, or standard 16G to 18G hypodermic needle) into the anteromedial surface of the proximal tibia ⅜" to 1¼" (1 to 3 cm) below the tibial tuberosity. To avoid the epiphyseal plate, direct the needle at a perpendicular or slightly inferior angle.

After penetrating the bony cortex and inserting the needle into the marrow cavity, you'll feel no resistance, you'll be able to aspirate bone marrow, the needle will remain upright without support, and the infusion will flow freely without subcutaneous infiltration. If bone or marrow obstructs the needle, replace the needle by passing a second one through the cannula.

When the needle is properly inserted, stabilize and secure it with gauze dressing and tape. Discontinue the intraosseous needle and line when a secure I.V. line is established.

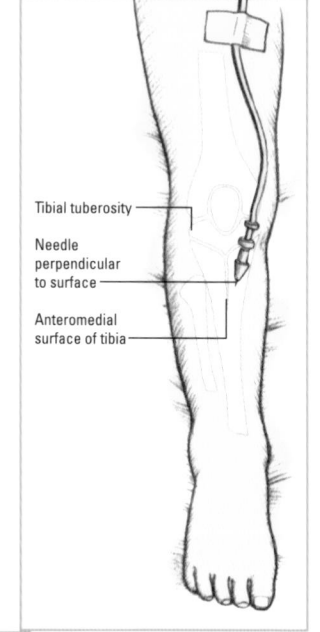

Tibial tuberosity

Needle perpendicular to surface

Anteromedial surface of tibia

Calculating pediatric fluid needs

Determining and meeting the fluid needs of children are important nursing responsibilities. Keep in mind that fluid replacement can also be affected by clinical conditions that cause fluid retention or loss. Children with these conditions should receive fluids based on their individual needs.

Fluid needs based on weight

• Children weighing under 10 kg require 100 ml of fluid per kilogram of body weight per day:

$$\text{weight in kg} \times 100 \text{ ml/kg/day} = \text{fluid needs in ml/day}$$

• Children weighing 10 to 20 kg require 1,000 ml of fluid per day for the first 10 kg plus 50 ml for every kilogram over 10:

$$(\text{total kg} - 10 \text{ kg}) \times 50 \text{ ml/kg/day} = \text{additional fluid need in ml/day}$$

$$1,000 \text{ ml/day} + \text{additional fluid need} = \text{fluid needs in ml/day}$$

• Children weighing more than 20 kg require 1,500 ml of fluid for the first 20 kg plus 20 ml for each additional kilogram:

$$(\text{total kg} - 20 \text{ kg}) \times 20 \text{ ml/kg/day} = \text{additional fluid need in ml/day}$$

$$1,500 \text{ ml/day} + \text{additional fluid need} = \text{fluid needs in ml/day}$$

Fluid needs based on calories

A child should receive 120 ml of fluid for every 100 kilocalories of metabolism (calorie requirements can be found in a table of recommended dietary allowances for children, or calculated by a dietitian):

$$\text{fluid requirements in ml/day} = \frac{\text{calorie requirements}}{100 \text{ kcal}} \times 120 \text{ ml}$$

Fluid needs based on BSA

Multiply the child's BSA by 1,500 to calculate the daily fluid needs of a child who isn't dehydrated:

$$\text{fluid maintenance needs in ml/day} = \text{BSA in m}^2 \times 1,500 \text{ ml/day/m}^2$$

I.V. insertion sites in infants

This illustration shows the preferred sites for inserting venous access devices in infants. If a scalp vein is used, hair may be shaved around the area to enable better visualization of the vein and monitoring of the site after insertion. (Be sure to prepare the parents for this possibility and save the hair for them.)

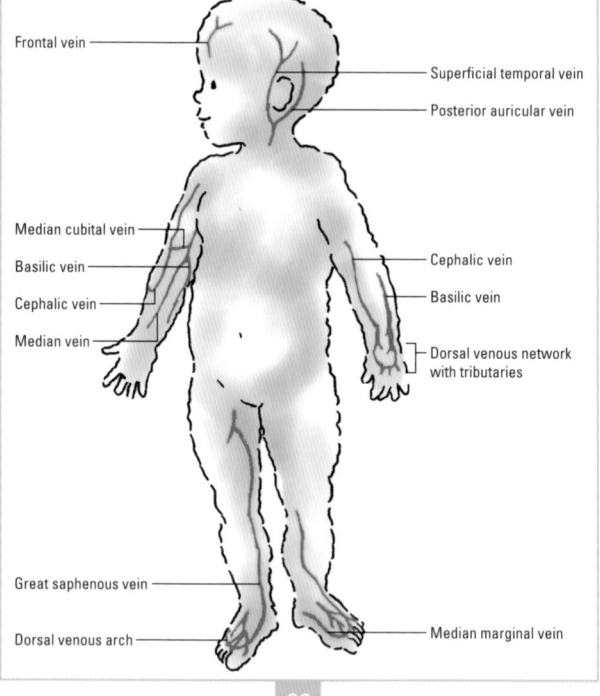

I.V. solutions

Isotonic

Isotonic solutions expand the intravascular compartment. When administering an isotonic solution, monitor for fluid overload. Isotonic solutions include:
• D_5W
• 0.9% NaCl
• Ringer's solution
• lactated Ringer's solution.

Hypertonic

Hypertonic solutions greatly expand the intravascular compartment and draw fluid from intravascular areas. When administering a hypertonic solution, monitor for fluid overload. Hypertonic solutions include:
• $D_{10}W$
• 3% NaCl
• 5% NaCl
• D_5LR
• D_5 0.45% NaCl
• D_5 0.9% NaCl.

Hypotonic

Hypotonic solutions cause a fluid shift from the intravascular compartment into the cells. When administering a hypotonic solution, monitor for cardiovascular collapse. Hypotonic solutions include:
• $D_{2.5}W$
• 0.45% NaCl
• 0.33% NaCl.

Determining compatibility for blood transfusions

		Compatible donors							
	(universal donor)	0–	0+	B–	B+	A–	A+	AB–	AB+
Patient's ABO group	(universal recipient) AB+	✓	✓	✓	✓	✓	✓	✓	✓
	AB–	✓		✓		✓		✓	
	A+	✓	✓			✓	✓		
	A–	✓				✓			
	B+	✓	✓	✓	✓				
	B–	✓		✓					
	0+	✓	✓						
	0–	✓							

Insulin overview

Insulin type	Onset	Peak	Usual effective duration	Usual maximum duration
Animal				
Regular	0.5 to 2 hr	3 to 4 hr	4 to 6 hr	6 to 8 hr
NPH	4 to 6 hr	8 to 14 hr	16 to 20 hr	20 to 24 hr
Human				
Insulin aspart	5 to 10 min	1 to 3 hr	3 to 5 hr	4 to 6 hr
Insulin lispro	< 15 min	0.5 to 1.5 hr	2 to 4 hr	4 to 6 hr
Regular	0.5 to 1 hr	2 to 3 hr	3 to 6 hr	6 to 10 hr
NPH	2 to 4 hr	4 to 10 hr	10 to 16 hr	14 to 18 hr
Lente	3 to 4 hr	4 to 12 hr	12 to 18 hr	16 to 20 hr
Ultralente	6 to 10 hr	—	18 to 20 hr	20 to 24 hr
Insulin glargine	1.1 hr	—	24 hr	24 hr

Insulin injection sites in children

Use these illustrations to instruct the child and his parents about the injection sites for insulin administration that are recommended by the American Diabetes Association.

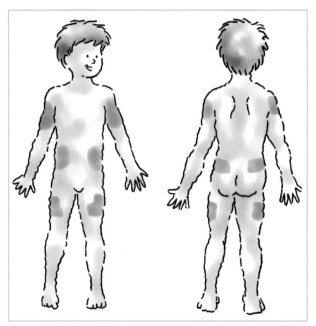

CPR

Infant (O to 1 year)

Check for unresponsiveness	Gently shake and flick bottom of foot and call out name.
Call for help/call 911	Call after 2 minutes of CPR; call immediately for witnessed collapse.
Position patient	Place patient in a supine position on a hard, flat surface.
Open airway	Use head-tilt, chin-lift maneuver unless contraindicated by trauma. Don't hyperextend the infant's neck.
If you suspect trauma	Open airway using jaw-thrust method if trauma is suspected.
Check breathing	Look, listen, and feel for 10 seconds.
Perform ventilations	Do two breaths at 1 second/breath initially; then one every 3 to 5 seconds.
If chest doesn't rise	Reposition and reattempt ventilation. Several attempts may be necessary.
Check pulse	Palpate brachial or femoral pulse for no more than 10 seconds.
Start compressions	
Placement	Place two fingers 1 fingerwidth below nipples.
Depth	⅓ to ½ depth of the chest
Rate	100/minute
Comp:Vent ratio	30:2 (If intubated, continuous chest compression at a rate of 100/min. without pauses for ventilation; ventilation at 8 to 10 breaths/min.)
Check pulse	Check after 2 minutes of CPR and as appropriate thereafter. Minimize interruptions in chest compressions.

CPR

Child (1 year to onset of adolescence or puberty)

Check for unresponsiveness	Gently shake and shout, "Are you okay?"
Call for help/call 911	Call after 2 min of CPR. Call immediately for witnessed collapse.
Position patient	Place patient in a supine position on a hard, flat surface.
Open airway	Use head-tilt, chin-lift maneuver unless contraindicated by trauma.
If you suspect trauma	Open airway using jaw-thrust method if trauma is suspected.
Check breathing	Look, listen, and feel for 10 sec.
Perform ventilations	Do two breaths initially that make the chest rise at 1 sec/breath; then one every 3 to 5 sec.
If chest doesn't rise	Reposition and reattempt ventilation. Several attempts may be necessary.
Check pulse	Palpate the carotid or femoral for no more than 10 sec.
Start compressions Placement	Place heel of one hand or place both hands, one atop the other, with elbows locked, on lower half of sternum between the nipples.
Depth	⅓ to ½ depth of the chest
Rate	100/min
Comp:Vent ratio	30:2 (if intubated, continuous chest compressions at a rate of 100/min without pauses for ventilation; ventilation at 8 to 10 breaths/min)
Check pulse	Check after 2 min of CPR and as appropriate thereafter. Minimize interruptions in chest compressions.
AED	Use as soon as available and follow prompts. Use child pads and child system for child age 1 to 8 years. Provide 2 min of CPR after first shock is delivered before activating AED to reanalyze rhythm and attempt another shock.

CPR

Before beginning basic life support, CPR, or rescue breathing, activate the appropriate code team.

Adolescent or adult

Check for unresponsiveness	Gently shake and shout, "Are you okay?"
Call for help/call 911	Immediately call 911 for help. If a second rescuer is available, send him to get help or an AED and initiate CPR if indicated. If asphyxial arrest is likely, perform 5 cycles (about 2 min) of CPR before activating EMS.
Position patient	Place patient in supine position on hard, flat surface.
Open airway	Use head-tilt, chin-lift maneuver unless contraindicated by trauma.
If you suspect trauma	Open airway using jaw-thrust method if trauma is suspected.
Check for adequate breathing	Look, listen, and feel for 10 sec.
Perform ventilations	Do two breaths initially that make the chest rise at 1 second/breath; then one every 5 to 6 sec.
If chest doesn't rise	Reposition and reattempt ventilation. Several attempts may be necessary.
Check pulse	Palpate the carotid for no more than 10 sec.
Start compressions	
Placement	Place both hands, one atop the other, on lower half of sternum between the nipples, with elbows locked; use straight up-and-down motion without losing contact with chest.
Depth	One-third depth of chest or 1½″ to 2″
Rate	100/min
Comp-to-vent ratio	30:2 (if intubated, continuous chest compressions at a rate of 100/min without pauses for ventilation; ventilation at 8 to 10 breaths/min)
Check pulse	Check after 2 min of CPR and as appropriate thereafter. Minimize interruptions in chest compressions.
Use AED	Apply as soon as available and follow prompts. Provide 2 min of CPR after first shock is delivered before activating AED to reanalyze rhythm and attempt another shock.

Choking

Infant (younger than 1 year)

Symptoms
- Inability to cry or make significant sound
- Weak, ineffective coughing
- Soft or high-pitched sounds while inhaling
- Bluish skin color

Interventions

1. Assess that airway is obstructed. *Don't* perform the next two steps if infant is coughing forcefully or has a strong cry.

2. Lay infant face down along your forearm. Hold infant's chest in your hand and his jaw with your fingers. Point the infant's head downward, lower than the body. Use your thigh or lap for support.

3. Give five quick, forceful blows between the infant's shoulder blades using the heel of your free hand.

After five blows

1. Turn the infant face up.

2. Place two fingers on the middle of infant's sternum just below the nipples.

3. Give five quick thrusts down, compressing the chest at ⅓ to ½ the depth of the chest or ½" to 1" (2 to 2.5 cm).

4. Continue five back blows and five chest thrusts until the object is dislodged or the infant loses consciousness. If the latter occurs, perform CPR. Each time you open the airway to deliver rescue breaths, look in the mouth and remove any object you see. Never perform a blind finger-sweep.

Choking

Child (older than 1 year) or adult

Symptoms

- Grabbing the throat with the hand
- Inability to speak
- Weak, ineffective coughing
- High-pitched sounds while inhaling

Interventions

1. Shout, "Are you choking? Can you speak?" Assess for airway obstruction. Don't intervene if the person is coughing forcefully and able to speak; a strong cough can dislodge the object.

2. Stand behind the person and wrap your arms around the person's waist (if pregnant or obese, wrap arms around chest).

3. Make a fist with one hand; place the thumbside of your fist just above the person's navel and well below the sternum.

4. Grasp your fist with your other hand.

5. Use quick, upward and inward thrusts with your fist (perform chest thrusts for pregnant or obese victims).

6. Continue thrusts until the object is dislodged or the victim loses consciousness. If the latter occurs, activate the emergency response number and provide CPR. Each time you open the airway to deliver rescue breaths, look in the mouth and remove any object you see. Never perform a blind finger-sweep.

Pediatric BLS algorithm

No movement or response

Send someone to phone 911; get AED.

Lone rescuer: For sudden collapse, phone 911 and get AED.

Open airway and check breathing.

If not breathing, give 2 breaths that make chest rise.

If no response, check pulse: Definite pulse within 10 seconds?

Definite pulse
- Give 1 breath every 3 seconds.
- Recheck pulse every 2 minutes.

No pulse

One rescuer: Give cycles of 30 compressions and 2 breaths. Push hard and fast (100/min) and release completely. Minimize interruptions in compressions.
Two rescuers: Give cycles of 15 compressions and 2 breaths.

If not already done, phone 911; for child, get AED/defibrillator.
Infant (<1 year): Continue CPR until ALS responders take over or victim starts to move.
Child (>1 year): Continue CPR; use AED/defibrillator after 5 cycles of CPR
(use AED as soon as it is available for sudden, witnessed collapse).

Give 1 shock. Resume CPR immediately for 5 cycles.

Shockable

Child > 1 year: Check rhythm. Shockable rhythm?

Not shockable

Resume CPR immediately for 5 cycles. Check rhythm every 5 cycles; continue until ALS providers take over or victim starts to move.

Source: American Heart Association. *Handbook of Emergency Cardiovascular Care for Healthcare Providers.* © 2006. Reproduced with permission.

Emergency

Pediatric pulseless arrest algorithm

1
Pulseless arrest
- BLS algorithm: Continue CPR.
- Give oxygen when available.
- Attach monitor/defibrillator when available.

3
VF/VT

Shockable

2
Check rhythm.
Shockable rhythm?

Not shockable

9
Asystole/PEA

4
Give 1 shock.
- Manual: 2 J/kg
- AED: >1 year of age
 Use pediatric system if available for 1 to 8 years of age.
  Resume CPR immediately.

Give 5 cycles of CPR. *

10
Resume CPR immediately.
 Give epinephrine.
- I.V./I.O.: 0.01 mg/kg (1:10000: 0.1 mL/kg)
- Endotracheal tube: 0.1 mg/kg
 (1:1000: 0.1 mL/kg)
  Repeat every 3 to 5 min.

Give 5 cycles of CPR. *

5
Check rhythm.
Shockable rhythm?

Not shockable

12
- If asystole, go to box 10.
- If electrical activity, check pulse. If no pulse, go to box 10.
- If pulse present, begin postresuscitation care.

Not shockable

11
Check rhythm.
Shockable rhythm?

Shockable

Shockable

6
Continue CPR while defibrillator is charging.
 Give 1 shock.
- Manual: 4 J/kg
- AED: >1 year of age
 Resume CPR immediately.
  Give epinephrine.
- I.V./I.O.: 0.01 mg/kg
 (1:10000: 0.1 mL/kg)
- Endotracheal tube:
 0.1 mg/kg (1:1000: 0.1 mL/kg)
 Repeat every 3 to 5 minutes.

13
Go to box 4

Give 5 cycles of CPR. *

7
Check rhythm.
Shockable rhythm?

Not shockable

Shockable

Shockable

8 Continue CPR while
defibrillator is charging.
Give 1 shock.
- Manual: 4 J/kg
- AED: >1 year of age
Resume CPR immediately.
Consider antiarrhythmics
(such as amiodarone
5 mg/kg I.V./I.O. or lidocaine
1 mg/kg I.V./I.O.).
Consider magnesium 25 to
50 mg/kg I.V./I.O., max 2 g for
torsades de pointes.
After 5 cycles of CPR*
go to box 5 above.

During CPR
- Push hard and fast (100/min).
- Ensure full chest recoil.
- Minimize interruptions in chest compressions.
- One cycle of CPR: 15 compressions, then 2 breaths;
  5 cycles ≈ 1 to 2 min.
- Avoid hyperventilation.
- Secure airway and confirm placement.
- Rotate compressors every 2 minutes with rhythm
  checks.
- Search for and treat possible contributing factors:

Hypovolemia
Hypoxia
Hydrogen ion (acidosis)
Hypokalemia or hyperkalemia
Hypoglycemia
Hypothermia
Toxins
Tamponade, cardiac
Tension pneumothorax
Thrombosis (coronary or pulmonary)
Trauma

* After an advanced airway is placed, rescuers no
longer deliver "cycles" of CPR. Give continuous chest
compressions without pauses for breaths. Give 8 to
10 breaths/minute. Check rhythm every 2 minutes.

Source: American Heart Association. *Handbook of Emergency Cardiovascular Care for Healthcare Providers.* © 2006. Reproduced with permission.

Pediatric tachycardia with pulses and poor perfusion algorithm

Tachycardia
with pulses and poor perfusion
- Assess and support ABCs as needed.
- Give oxygen.
- Attach monitor/defibrillator.

Symptoms persist

Evaluate QRS duration.

| **Narrow QRS (≤0.08 sec)** | **Wide QRS (>0.08 sec)** |

Evaluate rhythm with 12-lead ECG or monitor.

Possible ventricular tachycardia

Probable sinus tachycardia
- Compatible history consistent with known cause
- P waves present/ normal
- Variable RR; constant PR
- *Infants:* rate usually < 220 bpm
- *Children:* rate usually < 180 bpm

Probable supraventricular tachycardia
- Compatible history (vague, nonspecific)
- P waves absent/ abnormal
- HR not variable
- History of abrupt rate changes
- *Infants:* rate usually ≥ 220 bpm
- *Children:* rate usually ≥ 180 bpm

Search for and treat cause.

Consider vagal maneuvers (no delays)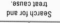

- Synchronized cardioversion: 0.5 to 1 J/kg; if not effective, increase to 2 J/kg
  Sedate if possible but don't delay cardioversion.
- May attempt adenosine if it doesn't delay electrical cardioversion.

94

- If I.V. access is readily available:
  Give adenosine 0.1 mg/kg (maximum first dose 6 mg) by rapid bolus.
  May double first dose and give once (maximum second dose 12 mg).

  OR

- Synchronized cardioversion: 0.5 to 1 J/kg; if not effective, increase to 2 J/kg. Sedate if possible but don't delay cardioversion.

Expert consultation advised
- Amiodarone 5 mg/kg I.V. over 20 to 60 minutes

  OR

- Procainamide 15 mg/kg I.V. over 30 to 60 minutes
  (Don't routinely administer amiodarone and procainamide together.)

During Evaluation
- Secure and verify airway and vascular access when possible.
- Consider expert consultation.
- Prepare for cardioversion.
  Treat possible contributing factors:
  Hypovolemia
  Hypoxia
  Hydrogen ion (acidosis)
  Hypokalemia or hyperkalemia
  Hypoglycemia
  Hypothermia
  Toxins
  Tamponade, cardiac
  Tension pneumothorax
  Thrombosis (coronary or pulmonary)
  Trauma (hypovolemia)

Emergency

Pediatric tachycardia with adequate perfusion algorithm

- BLS Algorithm: Assess and support ABCs (assess signs of circulation and pulse; provide oxygen and ventilation as needed).
- Provide oxygen.
- Attach monitor/defibrillator.
- Evaluate 12-lead ECG if practical.

What is the QRS duration?

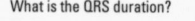

QRS normal (≤0.08 sec)

Evaluate rhythm.

QRS wide (>0.08 sec)

Probable ventricular tachycardia

Probable sinus tachycardia
- History compatible
- P waves present/normal
- HR often varies with activity
- Variable RR with constant PR
- *Infants:* rate usually <220 bpm
- *Children:* rate usually <180 bpm

Probable supraventricular tachycardia (ST)
- History incompatible with ST
- P waves absent/abnormal
- HR not variable with activity
- Abrupt rate changes
- *Infants:* rate usually ≥220 bpm
- *Children:* rate usually ≥180 bpm

Consider
alternative
medications.
- Amiodarone
5 mg/kg I.V.
over 30 to 60
minutes
  OR
- Procainamide
15 mg/kg I.V.
over 30 to 60
minutes
(Don't routinely
administer
amiodarone and
procainamide
together.)
  OR
- Lidocaine
1 mg/kg
I.V. bolus

Consider vagal
maneuvers

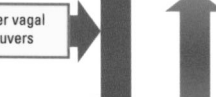

- Establish vascular access.
- Consider adenosine 0.1 mg/kg I.V. (maximum first dose: 6 mg).
- May double and repeat dose once (maximum second dose: 12 mg).
- Use rapid bolus technique.

During evaluation
- Provide oxygen and ventilation as needed.
- Support ABCs.
- Confirm continuous monitor/pacer attached.
- Consider expert consultation.
- Prepare for cardioversion 0.5 to 1 J/kg (consider sedation).

Identify and treat possible causes
- Hypovolemia
- Hypoxia
- Hyperthermia
- Hyperkalemia or hypokalemia and metabolic disorders
- Tamponade, cardiac
- Tension pneumothorax
- Toxins
- Thrombosis (coronary or pulmonary)
- Pain

- Consult pediatric cardiologist.
- Attempt cardioversion with 0.5 to 1 J/kg (may increase to 2 J/kg if initial dose is ineffective).
- Sedate prior to cardioversion.
- Obtain 12-lead ECG.

Emergency

Pediatric bradycardia with pulse algorithm

Bradycardia with a pulse causing cardiorespiratory compromise

↓

- Support ABCs as needed.
- Give oxygen.
- Attach monitor/defibrillator.

↓

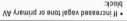

Bradycardia still causing cardiorespiratory compromise?

No →
- Support ABCs; give oxygen if needed.
- Observe.
- Consider expert consultation.

Yes ↓

Perform CPR if, despite oxygenation and ventilation, HR < 60/min with poor perfusion.

↓

Persistent symptomatic bradycardia?

No → (to box above)

Yes ↓

- Give epinephrine.
  - I.V./I.O.: 0.01 mg/kg (1:10000: 0.1 mL/kg)
  - Endotracheal tube: 0.1 mg/kg (1:1000: 0.1 mL/kg)
  - Repeat every 3 to 5 minutes.
- If increased vagal tone or primary AV block:
  - Give atropine, first dose: 0.02 mg/kg, may repeat. (Minimum dose: 0.1 mg; maximum total dose for child: 1 mg)
- Consider cardiac pacing.

↓

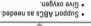

If pulseless arrest develops, go to Pulseless Arrest Algorithm.

SIDS prevention

Sudden infant death syndrome (SIDS) is the sudden death of a previously healthy infant when the cause of death isn't confirmed by a postmortem examination. It's the most common cause of death between ages 1 month and 1 year, and the third leading cause of death in all infants from birth to age 1 year. Even so, the incidence of SIDS has declined dramatically by more than 40% since 1992, which is mostly attributed to the 1992 initiative to put babies on their backs for sleeping, called the "Back to Sleep" campaign.

Preventive strategies

Parents should be informed of simple measures that they can take to prevent SIDS, including:
• putting the infant on his back to sleep
• not smoking anywhere near the infant
• removing from the infant's crib or sleeping environment all pillows, quilts, stuffed toys, and other soft surfaces that may trap exhaled air
• using a firm mattress with a snug-fitting sheet
• making sure the infant's head remains uncovered while sleeping
• keeping the infant warm while sleeping but not overheated.

Handling temper tantrums

As they assert their independence, toddlers demonstrate "temper tantrums," or violent objections to rules or demands. These tantrums include such behaviors as lying on the floor and kicking feet, screaming, or holding breath.

How to handle them

Dealing with a child's temper tantrums can be a challenge for parents who may be frustrated, embarrassed, or exhausted by their child's behavior. Reassure the parents that temper tantrums are a normal occurrence in toddlers, and that the child will outgrow them as he learns to express himself in more productive ways. This type of reassurance should be accompanied by some concrete suggestions for dealing effectively with temper tantrums:

• Provide a safe, childproof environment.
• Hold the child to keep him safe if his behavior is out of control.
• Give the toddler frequent opportunities to make developmentally appropriate choices.
• Give the child advance warning of a request to help prevent tantrums.
• Remain calm and be supportive of a child having a tantrum.
• Ignore tantrums when the toddler is seeking attention or trying to get something he wants.
• Help the toddler find acceptable ways to vent his anger and frustration.

When to get help

Parents should be advised to seek help from a health care provider when problematic tantrums:
• persist beyond age 5
• occur more than five times per day
• occur with a persistent negative mood
• cause property destruction
• cause harm to the child or others.

Choking hazards

Choking can easily occur in toddlers because they're still exploring their environments with their mouths. Toddlers may ingest small objects, while the small size of their oral cavities increases the risk of choking while eating. Foods that are round and less than 1" (2.5 cm) in diameter can obstruct the airway of a child when swallowed whole.

Common items that may cause choking include:
• foods, such as popcorn, peanuts, whole grapes, cherry or grape tomatoes, chunks of hot dogs, raw carrots, hard candy, bubble gum, long noodles, dried beans, and marshmallows
• small toys, such as broken latex balloons, button eyes, beaded necklaces, and small wheels
• common household items, such as broken zippers, pills, bottle caps, and nails and screws.

Preventive strategies

Provide parents with these preventive strategies to reduce the risk of choking:
• Cut food into small pieces to prevent obstruction of the airway. Slicing hot dogs into short, lengthwise pieces is a safe option.
• Avoid fruits with pits, fish with bones, hard candy, chewing gum, nuts, popcorn, whole grapes, and marshmallows.
• Encourage the child to sit whenever eating.
• Keep easily aspirated objects out of a toddler's environment.
• Be especially cautious about what toys the child plays with (choose sturdy toys without small, removable parts).
• Learn how to relieve airway obstruction in infants and children as part of a CPR course.

Toilet training

Physical readiness for toilet training occurs between ages 18 and 24 months; however, many children aren't cognitively ready to begin toilet training until they're between ages 36 and 42 months.

Signs of readiness

When physically and cognitively ready, the child can start toilet training. The process can take 2 weeks to 2 months to complete successfully. It's important to remember that there's considerable variation from one child to another. Other signs of readiness include:
• periods of dryness for 2 hours or more, indicating bladder control
• child's ability to walk well and remove clothing
• cognitive ability to understand the task
• facial expression or words suggesting that the child knows when he's about to defecate.

Step-by-step

Steps to toilet training include:
• teaching words for voiding and defecating
• teaching the purpose of the toilet or potty chair
• changing the toddler's diapers frequently to give him the experience of feeling dry and clean
• helping the toddler make the connection between dry pants and the toilet or potty chair
• placing the child on the potty chair or toilet for a few moments at regular intervals, and rewarding successes
• helping the toddler understand the physiologic signals by pointing out behaviors he displays when he needs to void or defecate
• rewarding successes but not punishing failures.

Preventing burns

Burns can easily occur in young children because they're tall enough to reach the stovetop and can walk to a fireplace or a wood stove to touch. Preventive measures to teach parents include:

• setting the hot water heater thermostat at a temperature less than 120° F (49° C)

• checking bath water temperature before a child enters the tub

• keeping pot handles turned inward and using the back burners on the stovetop

• keeping electrical appliances toward the backs of counters

• placing burning candles, incense, hot foods, and cigarettes out of reach

• avoiding the use of tablecloths so the curious child doesn't pull it to see what's on the table (possibly spilling hot foods or liquids on himself)

• teaching the child what "hot" means and stressing the danger of open flames

• storing matches and cigarette lighters in locked cabinets, out of reach

• burning fires in fireplaces or wood stoves with close supervision and using a fire screen when doing so

• securing safety plugs in all unused electrical outlets and keeping electrical cords tucked out of reach

• teaching preschoolers who can understand the hazards of fire to "stop, drop, and roll" if their clothes are on fire

• practicing escapes from home and school with preschoolers

• visiting a fire station to reinforce learning

• teaching preschoolers how to call 911 (for emergency use only).

Preventing poisoning

As a young child's gross motor skills improve and he becomes more curious, he's able to climb onto chairs and reach cabinets where medicines, cosmetics, cleaning products, and other poisonous substances are stored. Preventive measures to teach parents include:

• keeping medicines and other toxic materials locked away in high cupboards, boxes, or drawers
• using child-resistant containers and cupboard safety latches
• avoiding storage of a large supply of toxic agents
• teaching the child that medication isn't candy or a treat (even though it might taste good)
• teaching the child that plants inside or outside aren't edible, and keeping houseplants out of reach
• promptly discarding empty poison containers and never reusing them to store a food item or other poison
• always keeping original labels on containers of toxic substances
• having the poison control center number (1-800-222-1222) prominently displayed on every telephone. (The American Academy of Pediatrics no longer recommends keeping syrup of ipecac in the home; instead, parents should keep the poison control center number clearly posted.)

Preventing drowning

Toddlers and preschoolers are quite susceptible to drowning because they can walk onto docks or pool decks and stand or climb on seats in a boat. Drowning can also occur in mere inches of water, resulting from falls into buckets, bathtubs, hot tubs, toilets, and even fish tanks. Preventive strategies to teach parents include:

• instituting close adult supervision of any child near water
• teaching children never to go into water without an adult and never to horseplay near the water's edge
• using child-resistant pool covers and fences with self-closing gates around backyard pools
• emptying buckets when not in use and storing them upside-down
• using U.S. Coast Guard–approved child life jackets near water and on boats
• providing the child with swimming lessons.

Preventing falls

Falls can easily occur in young children as gross motor skills improve and they're able to move chairs to climb onto counters, climb ladders, and open windows. Preventive strategies to teach parents include:

• providing close supervision at all times during play
• keeping crib rails up and the mattress at the lowest position
• placing gates across the tops and bottoms of stairways
• installing window locks on all windows to keep them from opening more than 3″ (7.6 cm) without adult supervision

• keeping doors locked or using child-proof doorknob covers at entries to stairs, high porches or decks, and laundry chutes
• removing unsecured scatter rugs
• using a nonskid bath mat or decals in the bathtub or shower
• avoiding the use of walkers, especially near stairs
• always restraining children in shopping carts and never leaving them unattended
• providing safe climbing toys and choosing play areas with soft ground cover and safe equipment.

Motor vehicle and bicycle safety

Motor vehicle and bicycle injuries can easily occur in children because they may be able to unbuckle seat belts, resist riding in a car seat, or refuse to wear a bicycle helmet. Preventive measures to teach parents include:

• learning about the proper fit and use of bicycle helmets, and requiring the child to wear a helmet every time he rides a bicycle

• teaching the preschool-age child never to go into a road without an adult

• not allowing the child to play on a curb or behind a parked car

• checking the area behind vehicles before backing out of the driveway (small children may not be visible in rear-view mirrors because of blind spots, especially in larger vehicles)

• providing a safe, preferably enclosed, area for outdoor play for younger children (and keeping fences, gates, and doors locked)

• learning how to use child safety seats for all motor vehicle trips, and ensuring proper use by having the seats inspected (many local fire departments offer free inspections)

• encouraging older children to wear brightly colored clothing whenever riding bicycles. (Discourage the child from riding his bicycle during dusk hours or after dark; if he must ride during these hours, affix reflective tape to his clothing to make him easily visible and make sure his bicycle has a light and reflectors.)

Car safety seat guidelines

Proper installation and use of a car safety seat are critical. In addition to the weight and age guidelines outlined in the chart below, these guidelines for booster seat use will help ensure a child's safety while riding in a vehicle:

• Always make sure belt-positioning booster seats are used with both lap and shoulder belts.

• Make sure the lap belt fits low and right across the lap/upper thigh area and the shoulder belt fits snug, crossing the chest and shoulder to avoid abdominal injuries.

• All children younger than age 12 should ride in the back seat.

Weight and age	Seat type	Seat position
Up to 1 year or 20 lb	Infant-only or rear-facing convertible	Rear-facing
Up to 1 year and over 20 lb	Rear-facing convertible	Rear-facing
Over 1 year and 20 to 40 lb	Rear-facing convertible (until meeting seat manufacturer's limit for maximum weight and height), then forward-facing	Forward-facing
4 to 8 years and over 40 lb	Booster seat	Forward-facing

Neonate and infant weight conversion

Use this table to convert from pounds and ounces to grams when weighing neonates or infants.

Pounds	Ounces															
	0	1	2	3	4	5	6	7	8	9	10	11	12	13	14	15
0	—	28	57	85	113	142	170	198	227	255	283	312	340	369	397	425
1	454	484	510	539	567	595	624	652	680	709	737	765	794	822	850	879
2	907	936	964	992	1021	1049	1077	1106	1134	1162	1191	1219	1247	1276	1304	1332
3	1361	1389	1417	1446	1474	1503	1531	1559	1588	1616	1644	1673	1701	1729	1758	1786
4	1814	1843	1871	1899	1928	1956	1984	2013	2041	2070	2098	2126	2155	2183	2211	2240
5	2268	2296	2325	2353	2381	2410	2438	2466	2495	2523	2551	2580	2608	2637	2665	2693
6	2722	2750	2778	2807	2835	2863	2892	2920	2948	2977	3005	3033	3062	3090	3118	3147
7	3175	3203	3232	3260	3289	3317	3345	3374	3402	3430	3459	3487	3515	3544	3572	3600
8	3629	3657	3685	3714	3742	3770	3799	3827	3856	3884	3912	3941	3969	3997	4026	4054
9	4082	4111	4139	4167	4196	4224	4252	4281	4309	4337	4366	4394	4423	4451	4479	4508
10	4536	4564	4593	4621	4649	4678	4706	4734	4763	4791	4819	4848	4876	4904	4933	4961
11	4990	5018	5046	5075	5103	5131	5160	5188	5216	5245	5273	5301	5330	5358	5386	5415
12	5443	5471	5500	5528	5557	5585	5613	5642	5670	5698	5727	5755	5783	5812	5840	5868
13	5897	5925	5953	5982	6010	6038	6067	6095	6123	6152	6180	6209	6237	6265	6294	6322
14	6350	6379	6407	6435	6464	6492	6520	6549	6577	6605	6634	6662	6690	6719	6747	6776
15	6804	6832	6860	6889	6917	6945	6973	7002	7030	7059	7087	7115	7144	7172	7201	7228

Weight conversion

To convert a patient's weight in pounds to kilograms, divide the number of pounds by 2.2 kg; to convert a patient's weight in kilograms to pounds, multiply the number of kilograms by 2.2 lb.

Pounds	Kilograms
10	4.5
20	9
30	13.6
40	18.1
50	22.7
60	27.2
70	31.8
80	36.3
90	40.9
100	45.4
110	49.9
120	54.4
130	59
140	63.5
150	68
160	72.6
170	77.1
180	81.6
190	86.2
200	90.8
210	95.5
220	100
230	104.5
240	109.1
250	113.6
260	118.2
270	122.7
280	127.3
290	131.8
300	136.4

Temperature conversion

To convert Fahrenheit to Celsius, subtract 32 from the temperature in Fahrenheit and then divide by 1.8; to convert Celsius to Fahrenheit, multiply the temperature in Celsius by 1.8 and then add 32.

$$(F - 32) \div 1.8 = \text{degrees Celsius}$$

$$(C \times 1.8) + 32 = \text{degrees Fahrenheit}$$

Degrees Fahrenheit (°F)	Degrees Celsius (°C)	Degrees Fahrenheit (°F)	Degrees Celsius (°C)
89.6	32	100.8	38.2
91.4	33	101	38.3
93.2	34	101.2	38.4
94.3	34.6	101.4	38.6
95	35	101.8	38.8
95.4	35.2	102	38.9
96.2	35.7	102.2	39
96.8	36	102.6	39.2
97.2	36.2	102.8	39.3
97.6	36.4	103	39.4
98	36.7	103.2	39.6
98.6	37	103.4	39.7
99	37.2	103.6	39.8
99.3	37.4	104	40
99.7	37.6	104.4	40.2
100	37.8	104.6	40.3
100.4	38	104.8	40.4
		105	40.6

Nutritional guidelines for infants and toddlers

• Breast-feeding is recommended exclusively for the first 6 months of life, and then should be continued in combination with infant foods until age 1 year.

• If breast-feeding isn't possible or desired, bottle-feeding with iron-fortified infant formula is an acceptable alternative for the first 12 months of life.

• After age 1, whole cow's milk can be used in place of breast milk or formula.

• New foods should be introduced to the infant's diet one at a time, waiting 5 to 7 days between them. If the infant rejects a food initially, the parents should offer it again later.

• Unpasteurized products, such as honey or corn syrup, should be avoided.

• Toddlers should be offered a variety of foods, including plenty of fruits, vegetables, and whole grains.

• Serving size should be approximately 1 tablespoon of solid food per year of age (or one-fourth to one-third the adult portion size) so as not to overwhelm the child with larger portions.

Solid foods and infant age

Age	Type of food	Rationale
4 mo	Rice cereal mixed with breast milk or formula	Are less likely than wheat to cause an allergic reaction
5 to 6 mo	Strained vegetables (offered first) and fruits	Offer first because they may be more readily accepted than if introduced after sweet fruits
7 to 8 mo	Strained meats, cheese, yogurt, rice, noodles, pudding	Provide an important source of iron and add variety to the diet
8 to 9 mo	Finger foods (bananas, crackers)	Promote self-feeding
10 mo	Mashed egg yolk (no whites until age 1); bite-size cooked food (no foods that may cause choking)	Decrease risk of choking (avoiding foods that can cause choking is the safest option, even though the infant chews well)
12 mo	Foods from the adult table (chopped or mashed according to the infant's ability to chew foods)	Provide a nutritious and varied diet that should meet the infant's nutritional needs

Nutritional guidelines for children older than age 2 years

Key recommendations for children and adolescents from the Dietary Guidelines for Americans (2005) issued by the U.S. Department of Health and Human Services and the U.S. Department of Agriculture are listed here. All children should be encouraged to eat a variety of fruits, vegetables, and whole grains.

Weight management

• For overweight children and adolescents, reduce body weight gain while achieving normal growth and development. Consult with a health care practitioner before placing a child on a weight-reduction diet.

• For overweight children with chronic diseases or those on medication, consult with a health care practitioner before starting a weight-reduction program to ensure management of other health conditions.

Physical activity

• Children and adolescents should engage in at least 60 minutes of physical activity on most, preferably all, days.

Food groups to encourage

• At least one-half of grains consumed should be whole grains.

• Children ages 2 to 8 years should consume 2 cups of fat-free or low-fat milk (or equivalent milk product) per day.

• Children ages 9 years and older should consume 3 cups of fat-free or low-fat milk (or equivalent milk product) per day.

Fats

• For children ages 2 to 3 years, fat intake should be 30% to 35% of total daily calories consumed.

• For children ages 4 to 18 years, fat intake should be 25% to 35% of total daily calories consumed.

• Most fats should come from sources of polyunsaturated and monounsaturated fatty acids, such as fish, nuts, and vegetable oils.

Food safety

• Infants and young children shouldn't eat or drink raw (unpasteurized) milk or products made from unpasteurized milk, raw or partially cooked eggs or foods containing raw eggs, raw or undercooked meat or poultry, raw or uncooked fish or shellfish, unpasteurized juices, or raw sprouts.

Preventing obesity

Obesity and overweight have become serious health problems. An estimated 16% of children and adolescents are now overweight. Over the last two decades, this rate has skyrocketed in young Americans; the rate has doubled in children and tripled in adolescents. Excess body fat is problematic because it increases a person's risk for developing such serious health problems as type 2 diabetes, hypertension, dyslipidemia, certain types of cancers, and more. Additionally, overweight children have a high probability of becoming obese adults.

What to do

Weight-loss diets may not be the answer for children and adolescents because growth and development increase nutritional needs. However, some dietary changes can have significant results. Suggestions include:
• avoiding fast-food
• eating low-fat after-school snacks
• switching from whole milk to skim milk
• exchanging fresh vegetables for fried snack foods
• eating a variety of fresh and dried fruits.

Additionally, children who are overweight or even of normal weight should be encouraged to participate in some type of daily vigorous, aerobic activity to help reduce or prevent childhood obesity and promote a habit of daily exercise that will last a lifetime.

Healthy snacks for children

Encourage parents of your pediatric patients to begin good eating habits early by offering healthy snacks to their children. Here are some suggestions:
• peanut butter spread on apple slices or rice cakes
• frozen yogurt topped with berries or fruit slices
• raw or dried fruit served with a dip such as low-fat yogurt or pudding
• raw red and green peppers, carrots, and celery sticks served with low-fat salad dressing as a dip
• fruit smoothies made with blended low-fat milk or yogurt and fresh or frozen fruit
• applesauce.

The Food Guide Pyramid

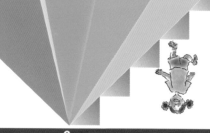

*

Grains	Vegetables	Fruits	Milk	Meat and Beans
An ounce equivalent is: — 1 slice of bread — ½ cup of cooked cereal like oatmeal — ½ cup of rice or pasta — 1 cup cold cereal • 4- to 8-year-olds need 4- to 5-ounce equivalents/day. • 9- to 13-year-old girls need 5-ounce equivalents/day. • 9- to 13-year-old boys need 6-ounce equivalents/day.	• 4- to 8-year-olds need 1½ cups/day. • 9- to 13-year-old girls need 2 cups/day. • 9- to 13-year-old boys need 2½ cups/day.	• 4- to 8-year-olds need 1 to 1½ cups/day. • 9- to 13-year-olds need 1½ cups/day.	(or other calcium-rich foods such as yogurt, cheese, or calcium-fortified orange juice for example) — 1 cup • 2- to 3-year-olds need 2 cups/day (or other calcium-rich foods). • 4- to 8-year-olds need 2 cups/day (or other calcium-rich foods). • 9- to 13-year-olds need 3 cups/day (or other calcium-rich foods).	An ounce equivalent is: — 1 oz of meat, poultry, or fish — ¼ cup dry beans cooked — 1 egg — 1 table-spoon of peanut butter — small handful of nuts or seeds. • 4- to 13-year-olds need 5½-ounce equivalents/day.

Fats *

• 2- to 3-year-olds need 30% to 35% of total daily calories to come from fat.
• 4- to 18-year-olds need 25% to 35% of total daily calories to come from fat.

Most fat should come from fish, nuts, and vegetable oils.

Adapted from U.S. Department of Agriculture, Center for Nutrition Policy and Promotion, April 2005. Available at www.mypyramid.gov.

114

Sleep guidelines

Age-group	Hrs of sleep needed per day	Special considerations
Infant		
Birth to 6 mo	15 to 16½	• To help prevent sudden infant death syndrome, all infants should be placed on their backs to sleep.
6 mo to 12 mo	13¾ to 14½	• At ages 4 to 6 months, infants are physiologically capable of sleeping (without feeding) for 6 to 8 hours at night.
		• From birth to age 3 months, infants may take many naps per day; from ages 4 to 9 months, two naps per day; and by 9 to 12 months, only one nap per day.
Toddler		
1 to 2 yr	10 to 15	• Most toddlers sleep through the night without awakening.
2 to 3 yr	10 to 12	• A consistent routine (set bedtime, reading, and a security object) helps toddlers prepare for sleep.
		• Up to age 3, toddlers take one nap per day; after age 3, many toddlers don't need a nap.
Preschool-age	10 to 12	• If the preschooler no longer naps, a "quiet" or rest period may be useful.
		• Dreams or nightmares become more real as magical thinking increases and a vivid imagination develops.
		• Problems falling asleep may occur due to over-stimulation, separation anxiety, or fear of the dark or monsters.
School-age	9 to 10	• Compliance at bedtime becomes easier.
		• Nightmares are usually related to a real event in the child's life and can usually be eradicated by resolving any underlying fears the child might have.
		• Sleepwalking and sleeptalking may begin.
Adolescent	At least 8	• Sleep requirements increase because of physical growth spurts and high activity levels.
		• The hours needed for sleep can't be made up or stored ("catch-up" sleep on the weekends isn't effective in replenishing a teen's sleep store).

Resources

Cultural considerations in patient care

As a health care professional you'll interact with a diverse, multicultural patient population. Each culture has its own unique set of beliefs about health and illness and dietary practices that you need to know when providing care.

Cultural group	Health and illness philosophy	Dietary practices
African Americans	• May believe illness is related to supernatural causes, such as punishment from God or an evil spell • May express grief by crying, screaming, praying, singing, and reading scripture • May seek advice and remedies from faith or folk healers	• May have food restrictions based on religious beliefs, such as not eating pork if Muslim • May view cooked greens as good for health
Arab Americans	• Believe health is a gift from God and that one should care for self by eating right and minimizing stressors • If devout, may interpret illness as the will of Allah or a test of faith and, therefore, have a fatalistic view • Believe in complete rest and relieving self of all responsibilities during an illness • May express pain freely • After death, may want to prepare the body by washing it and then wrapping it in a white cloth • Discourage postmortem examination unless required by law	• Don't mix sweet and sour or hot and cold • Don't use ice in drinks; believe hot soup can help recovery • If Muslim, prohibited from drinking alcohol and eating pork or ham

Cultural considerations in patient care

(continued)

Cultural group	Health and illness philosophy	Dietary practices
Chinese Americans	• Believe health is a balance of Yin and Yang and illness stems from an imbalance of these elements; health requires harmony between body, mind, and spirit • May use herbalists or acupuncturists before seeking medical help • May use good luck objects, such as jade or a rope tied around the waist • Family expected to take care of the patient, who assumes a passive role • Tend not to readily express pain; stoic by nature	• Staples are rice, noodles, and vegetables; tend to use chopsticks • Choose foods to help balance the Yin (cold) and Yang (hot) • Drink hot liquids, especially when sick
Japanese Americans	• Believe that health is a balance of oneself, society, and the universe • May believe illness is karma, resulting from behavior in present or past life • May believe certain food combinations cause illness • May not complain of symptoms until severe	• Eat rice with most meals; may use chopsticks • Diet high in salt; low in sugar, fat, animal protein, and cholesterol

(continued)

Cultural considerations in patient care
(continued)

Cultural group	Health and illness philosophy	Dietary practices
Latino Americans	• May view illness as a sign of weakness, punishment for evil doing, or retribution for shameful behavior • May use the terms hot and cold in reference to vital elements needed to restore equilibrium to body • May consult with a curandero (healer) or voodoo preist (Caribbean) • May view pain as a necessary part of life and believe that enduring pain is a sign of strength (especially men) • May openly express grief, such as by praying for the dead or saying the rosary • May use amulets to ward off evil • Typically involve family members in all aspects of decision making, such as with terminal illness	• Beans and tortillas are staples • Eat lots of fresh fruits and vegetables
Native Americans	• Use herbs and roots; each tribe has its own unique medicinal practices • Most use modern medicine where available • Use Medicine Wheel, an ancient symbol • For some, 4 is a sacred number, associated with the four primary laws of creation: Life, Unity, Equality, and Eternity • May use tobacco for important religious, ceremonial, and medicinal purposes; may sprinkle it around the bed of sick people to protect and heal them • May believe that the spirit of a dying person can't leave the body until the family is present	• Have balanced diet of seafood, fruits, greens, corn, rice, and garden vegetables; salt consumption is low • Specific dietary practices are based on location; urban dwellers commonly eat most types of meat, while rural dwellers commonly consume only lamb and goat

Selected references

Bowden, V.R. "Get Involved! Join a Pediatric Nursing Association Just Right for You," *Pediatric Nursing* 29(5):397-402, September-October 2003.

Bowden, V.R., and Greenberg, C.S. *Pediatric Nursing Procedures.* Philadelphia: Lippincott Williams & Wilkins, 2003.

Boynton, R.W., et al. *Manual of Ambulatory Pediatrics,* 5th ed. Philadelphia: Lippincott Williams & Wilkins, 2003.

Fleitas, J. "The Power of Words: Examining the Linguistic Landscape of Pediatric Nursing," *MCN, The American Journal of Maternal/Child Nursing* 28(6):384-88, November-December 2003.

Godshall, M. "Caring for Families of Chronically Ill Kids," *RN* 66(2):30-35, February 2003.

Hockenberry, M.J., et al. *Wong's Nursing Care of Infants and Children,* 7th ed. St. Louis: Mosby–Year Book, Inc., 2003.

Hodges, E.A. "A Primer on Early Childhood Obesity and Parental Influence," *Pediatric Nursing* 29(1):13-16, January-February 2003.

Jakubik, L.D., et al. "The ABCs of Pediatric Laboratory Interpretation: Understanding the CBC with Differential and LFTs," *Pediatric Nursing* 29(2):97-103, March-April 2003.

Limbo, R., et al. "Promoting Safety of Young Children with Guided Participation Process," *Journal of Pediatric Health Care* 17(5):245-51, September-October 2003.

Link, N. "Keeping Kids Comfortable," *Nursing2003* 33(7):22, July 2003.

Mandleco, B. *Growth and Development Handbook: Newborn Through Adolescent.* Clifton Park, N.Y.: Delmar Learning, 2004.

Miaskowski, C. "Identifying Issues in the Management of Pain in Infants and Children," *Pain Management Nursing* 4(1):1-2, March 2003.

Pillitteri, A. *Maternal and Child Health Nursing: Care of the Childbearing and Childrearing Family,* 4th ed. Philadelphia: Lippincott Williams & Wilkins, 2003.

Rebeschi, L.M., and Brown, M.H. *The Pediatric Nurse's Survival Guide,* 2nd ed. Clifton Park, N.Y.: Delmar Learning, 2002.

Reed, P., et al. "Promoting the Dignity of the Child in Hospital," *Nursing Ethics* 10(1):67-76, January 2003.

Reyes, S. "Nursing Assessment of Infant Pain," *Journal of Perinatal and Neonatal Nursing* 17(4):291-303, October-November 2003.

Straight A's in Pediatric Nursing. Philadelphia: Lippincott Williams & Wilkins, 2004.

Story, M.T., et al. "Management of Child and Adolescent Obesity: Attitudes, Barriers, Skills, and Training Needs Among Health Care Professionals," *Pediatrics* 110(1 Pt 2):210-14, July 2002.

Taketomo, C.K., et al. *Pediatric Dosage Handbook,* 11th ed. Hudson, Ohio: Lexi-Comp, Inc., 2004.

Index